EPILEPSY 101

THE ULTIMATE GUIDE FOR PATIENTS AND FAMILIES

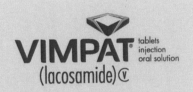

VIMPAT® tablets
injection
oral solution

(lacosamide) Ⓒ

Provided as an educational service by UCB

UCB, Inc. is proud to provide this medical book to you as an educational tool. The contents of this book were independently developed and do not necessarily reflect the ideas and beliefs of UCB. In addition, this book may contain discussions on uses of products that have not been approved by the FDA. Please refer to the attached product information for the approved uses and full safety information for UCB Products. This book does not replace the medical advice of a healthcare provider. No prescribing decisions should be made based on the contents of this book. UCB assumes no responsibility for any injury or damage to persons or property arising or related to any use of the material contained in this book.

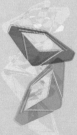

VE1135-0710D

EPILEPSY 101

THE ULTIMATE GUIDE FOR PATIENTS AND FAMILIES

by

The National Epilepsy Educational Alliance

Medicus Press

ISBN-13: 978-0-9787727-3-4

This publication is designed to provide accurate and authoritative information in regard to the subject matter covered. It is sold with the understanding that neither the author nor the publisher shall be liable or responsible for any loss, injury or damage allegedly arising from any information or suggestion in this book. The treatments, medicines, procedures and other suggestions contained in this book are not intended as a substitute for consulting with a physician. The reader should consult with a physician in matters relating to her/his health and particularly with respect to any symptoms that may require diagnosis or medical attention.

First Printing

To order visit www.medicuspress.com

Cover design:
Figure con Sol (Figure with Sun)
by Raul Vasquez Saenz 2003
Panamanian Painter (d. 2008)

To our patients and their families

CONTENTS

The National Epilepsy Educational Alliance

Ruben Kuzniecky, M.D., Chair

B. Abou-Khalil, M.D.

G. Barkley, M.D.

G. Cascino, M.D.

M. Duchowny, M.D.

E. Faught, M.D.

J. French, M.D.

J. Gates, M.D.

F. Gilliam M.D.

C. Harden, M.D.

A. Kanner, M.D.

P. Kotagal, M.D.

D. Lowenstein, M.D.

K. Meador, M.D.

D. Nordli, M.D.

S. Pacia, M.D.

P. Pennell, M.D.

R. Radke, M.D.

R. Sankar, M.D.

M. Sperling, M.D.

D. Treimann, M.D.

E. Vinning, M.D.

D. Vossler, M.D.

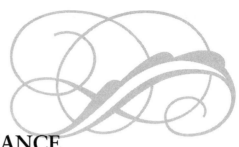

EPILEPSY EDUCATIONAL ALLIANCE

Contributors

Bassel Abou-Khalil, M.D.
Epilepsy Center
Vanderbilt University Medical Center
Nashville, Tennessee

Gregory Barkley, M.D.
Epilepsy Center
Henry Ford Hospital
Detroit, Michigan

Gregory Cascino, M.D.
Epilepsy Section
Mayo Clinic
Rochester, Minnesota

Michael Duchowny, M.D.
Epilepsy Center
Miami Children's Hospital
Miami, Florida

Edward Faught, M.D.
Epilepsy Center
University of Alabama
Birmingham, Alabama

Jacqueline French, M.D.
Epilepsy Center
New York University
New York, New York

John Gates, M.D.
Minnesota Epilepsy Group
St. Paul, Minnesota

Frank Gilliam, M.D.
Epilepsy Center
Weill Cornell Medical College
New York, New York

Cynthia Harden, M.D.
Epilepsy Center
University of Miami
Miami, Florida

Andres Kanner, M.D.
Epilepsy Center
Rush University Medical Center
Chicago, Illinois

Prakash Kotagal, M.D.
Epilepsy Center
Cleveland Clinic Foundation
Cleveland, Ohio

Ruben Kuzniecky, M.D.
Epilepsy Center
New York University
New York, New York

Daniel Lowenstein, M.D.
Epilepsy Center
University of California
  San Francisco
San Francisco, California

Kimford Meador, M.D.
Emory University
Atlanta, Georgia

Douglas Nordli, M.D.
Children's Memorial Hospital
Northwest University
Chicago, Illinois

Steven Pacia, M.D.
Epilepsy Center
New York University
New York, New York

Page Pennell, M.D.
Epilepsy Center
Brigham and Women's Hospital
Boston, Massachusetts

Rod Radke, M.D.
Epilepsy Center
Duke University Medical Center
Durham, North Carolina

Raman Sankar, M.D.
David Geffen School of Medicine
UCLA Epilepsy Center
Los Angeles, California

Michael Sperling, M.D.
Epilepsy Center
Thomas Jefferson University Hospital
Philadelphia, Pennsylvania

David Treiman, M.D.
Epilepsy Center
Barrow Neurological Institute
Phoenix, Arizona

Eileen Vining, M.D.
Epilepsy Center
John Hopkins Medical Institutions
Baltimore, Maryland

David Vossler, M.D.
Neuroscience Institute
Valley Medical Center
Renton, Washington

PREFACE

THE IMPETUS FOR THIS BOOK arose from an informal conversation among some of the authors at one of our medical meetings. The idea of a *common effort* arising from leading epilepsy specialists in the United States to create a patient guide and companion was highly attractive. All of those who contributed directly and indirectly felt from the onset that creating a balanced, comprehensive and informative guide would improve patient care. The idea of creating an epilepsy companion also arose from the findings that this type of guide does not exist for patients and families with epilepsy.

Caring for patients with epilepsy is challenging. Diagnosis, treatment, prognosis and genetics of seizures and epilepsy are complex and rapidly changing. Patients and families not only have to deal with the medical aspects of the disorder but more important, with the psychological, social and emotional impact of epilepsy in their daily lives.

This guide and workbook is intended to help patients and families learn about their condition and deal with many of the common non-medical aspects. It provides clear and basic information about the disorder, its diagnosis and the different treatment modalities available. This guide and companion also emphasizes emotional and social issues. The text is broadly based on the ideas and practices of a large group of epilepsy experts in the United States and thus, some aspects need to be viewed in this context. The book is also intended to be a workbook and companion. We have incorporated side-effect scales, seizure diaries and resource information in the hope that patients will use it during their medical visits.

In the end, this workbook, guide, and companion is intended to improve the quality of life of patients and families. We hope we have achieved what we set to do.

Ruben Kuzniecky, M.D.
Professor
NYU Epilepsy Center
New York University
New York

ACKNOWLEDGMENTS

WE ARE INDEBTED TO MANY people who contributed to this work. All of us depend on our office staff and nurses to help us care for our patients. Their time and efforts assisted us in having some free moments to write these pages. We are particularly indebted to George Lai and Anjanette Burns who read the manuscript, obtained figures and artwork and helped with many aspects. Without them, much of it would have not been possible. We also thank Meghan Fusz who contributed to Chapter 10.

We are grateful to Terry Blalock from Glaxo who supported this work with an unrestricted educational grant. We are also thankful to the staff of Medicus Press for enduring our protracted course, to Joann Woy and Patty Wallenburg for their book making expertise and to many others who made this work possible. Finally, and most importantly, to our patients. What we learn every-day from each of them is inspiring and humbling. We hope we have not disappointed any of them.

INTRODUCTION

EPILEPSY, SEIZURES, CONVULSIONS, attacks, spells, and falls; these are some of the most common terms we hear people use when dealing with epilepsy. Centuries of misunderstanding, demonization, and discrimination caused those with seizures and epilepsy to hide their burden in the closet. Fortunately, over the past 20 years, we have seen the gradual disappearance of these attitudes, to the great benefit of patients and families affected by epilepsy and seizures.

The word *epilepsy* is a general term that cannot be considered a disease or a diagnosis. To say that a person has epilepsy has no specific meaning, and it should not be considered a final diagnosis. While it may give a general indication of the nature of a problem, the term is so unspecific as to be almost meaningless in many ways. "Epilepsy" includes a large number of conditions that can manifest in many ways. Although this may seem complicated, a good way to gain a better understanding is to think about epilepsy in the same way we think about anemia (low blood count). Neither epilepsy nor anemia is a disease. Anemia can be caused by low blood iron, lack of vitamins, loss of blood, and more. Similarly, epilepsy and/or seizures can result from low sodium (salt) in your blood, abnormal genes, a blow to the head, a brain infection, a brain tumor, or other causes. A seizure is simply a manifestation of abnormal brain function (see Chapter 1).

The brain is the most complex and marvelous organ of the human body and thus is very sensitive to minor changes in function. If something goes wrong, the problem will manifest itself in abnormal functioning in various systems of the body, such as problems with vision, hearing, language, memory, behavior, and the like. In simpler terms, abnormal brain function can be exposed by either a loss of function or an excess of activity, due mostly to an imbalance between affected systems. For example, a stroke will destroy an area of brain tissue and result in a loss of function in that area. The most common case is a stroke victim who has lost the ability to use his arm and hand due to paralysis. On the other hand, seizures or epilepsy can also arise from too much abnormal activity in a brain region. The following chapters will explore in more detail all aspects of seizures and epilepsy.

HISTORICAL BACKGROUND

In the earliest writings, it was believed that epilepsy, also known as the "sacred disease," was caused by possession by evil spirits or gods. The word *epilepsy* is derived from the Greek verb *epil-*

amvanein, which means "to be seized," and is associated with possession by evil spirits. Treatment therefore involved the use of religious, occult, and magical powers—and some less than pleasant experiences. The Mesopotamian, Hebrew, and Egyptian civilizations knew of the disease for centuries. The Greek physicians of the Hippocrates school mentioned epilepsy as the sacred disease, despite the fact that the Greek's rejected the idea that epilepsy was a form of punishment inflicted by the gods. On the contrary, they believed that something in the brain was its cause. Even though they attempted to refute its connection to the supernatural, the treatment of epilepsy remained attached to charlatans, superstition, and magic powers for many centuries.

In the Middle Ages, fear of epilepsy and seizures became even more radical. People with epilepsy were accused of possessing devils and were targeted for death, which brought much destruction on many people, particularly women. If patients continued to have seizures despite exorcism, they were frequently put to death. Even at the end of the nineteenth century, it was possible for a reputable medical practitioner specializing in the treatment of epilepsy to advocate in a lecture in New York that various forms of mutilation were appropriate for the treatment of epilepsy—including castration because convulsions were believed to originate in the testes, and masturbation was believed to exacerbate epileptic seizures.

The modern view of epilepsy is generally considered to have originated with the studies and work of John Hughlings Jackson, an Englishman born in Yorkshire. In 1862, at the age of 27, Jackson was appointed as assistant physician to the National Hospital for the Relief and Cure of the Paralyzed and Epileptic (now the National Hospital for Neurology and Neurosurgery) Queen Square, London. As in many cases in medicine, Jackson had a close relationship with epilepsy—his wife developed motor seizures following a stroke. During the attacks, her hand began jerking, then her leg, then her face. This type of epilepsy, with its typical march of symptoms, became known as Jacksonian epilepsy. Since Jackson was puzzled by brain function, he used his observations to develop a view of neurology that related where functions were located in the brain. In 1873, Jackson presented his classic definition of epileptic seizures as "occasional sudden excessive, rapid, and local discharges of gray matter." This view established focal seizures as being truly epileptic in origin. The combination of scientific research and clinical findings enabled Jackson's ideas to be confirmed by other scientists performing experiments in animals. As a result, the first step of the modern era of epilepsy treatment began (see Chapters 1 and 2).

SEIZURE SURGERY

Using this incredible skill for brain localization and using the patient's complaints as a guide to the site of the seizure focus, in 1879, a neurosurgeon in Glasgow, William Macewen, correctly localized a brain tumor and undertook surgery to cure epilepsy. Following tumor removal, the patient survived and became seizure free. Almost simultaneously, in London, Jackson convinced a young neurosurgeon named Victor Horsley to operate on a young man who had frequent seizures due to a head injury caused by a horse kick. This case, in addition to a few others, represents the origin of neurosurgery for the treatment of epilepsy. Although these early cases were successful, establishing the principle of seizure control by surgical removal of the "seizure focus," the success of surgery for epilepsy was poor, and eventually operative treatment fell into disuse. Over time, discoveries and improvements in anesthesia, antisepsis, and antibiotics made a large impact on the safety of neurosurgery for epilepsy, just as they did in many other areas of medicine.

THE MODERN ERA

During the twentieth century, Wilder Penfield, who, in 1934, founded the Montreal Neurologic Institute at McGill University in Montreal, became the lead figure in furthering the development of the surgical treatment for epilepsy and the localization of brain function. In common with Jackson, his extensive writings, coupled with a clear, detailed, and objective skills in observation, provided a wealth of information that remains important to this day.

In 1929, Hans Berger, a German psychiatrist, published the technique of electroencephalogram (EEG) and showed for the first time that electrical activity of the brain could be recorded. Although Berger was disappointed that the EEG was of limited use in psychiatric patients, he showed that abnormal waves could be recorded in patients with seizures. Soon after his findings were confirmed, many centers around the world began using the EEG to study and treat patients with seizures. This important technology was further developed by many researchers to provide a means to localize those areas of the brain where seizures originated. This was a very exciting time in neurology since, for the first time ever, physicians had a real test that could be used not only to find the area in the brain that caused seizures but also to separate different seizure types. In 1934, in Boston, Dr. Frederick Gibbs showed the spike-and-wave EEG pattern of "petite mal" for the first time and, a few years later, Dr. Herbert Jasper worked with Wilder Penfield in Montreal to use the EEG to help in the surgical treatment of certain epilepsies. EEG technology developed to the point where, in 1951, P. Bailey, a neurosurgeon in Chicago, published a paper documenting a series of patients who had temporal lobe surgery based *only* on EEG alone. The results were encouraging and helped established the EEG as the prime method to study seizures. Over the next 30 years, the study of epilepsy was dominated by the technical development and understanding of the information obtained from the EEG. During this period, surgery, as a treatment of epilepsy, also gained considerable ground.

A MORE MODERN VIEW OF EPILEPSY AND SEIZURES

As we enter the twenty-first century, we have gained much knowledge about epilepsy and seizures. No longer are patients hidden from society; we now know and understand that epilepsy is not an "untouchable" disorder. Additionally, we have many new diagnostic test, medications, and better surgical techniques. In particular, modern imaging techniques, such as magnetic resonance imaging (MRI), have had an impact as large as that of EEG more than 70 years ago. In this day and age, we are now entering the genetic era of epilepsy as we try to solve the puzzles of why, what, and how epilepsy occurs. What has become clear over time, however, is that no single mechanism or cause underlies all epilepsies. Therefore, treatment of seizures and epilepsy is likely to change even more in the years to come.

1

EPILEPSY AND SEIZURES

An Overview

Key Points

▶ A *seizure* is what happens when the brain has abnormal, uncontrolled electrical activity.

▶ *Epilepsy* is used to describe a condition in which a person has a tendency for recurrent seizures.

▶ There are about 10 billion neurons in the human brain.

▶ Focal seizures come from a discrete *focus* in the brain.

▶ An aura can occur as a stand-alone event, but it often progresses into a complex focal seizure.

▶ Probably the most commonly recognized seizure type is the tonic–clonic (or *grand mal*) seizure.

▶ *Myoclonic seizures* refer to extremely brief, jerking movements.

▶ The most common example of a symptomatic localization-related epilepsy occurs in *temporal lobe epilepsy.*

▶ Epilepsy is widely thought to be a disorder of childhood, but it is common at any age.

Defining Some Basic Terms

Before getting into a description of what goes on in the brain when a person has a seizure, it is important to first be clear about the definitions of words such as "seizure" and "epilepsy." A *seizure* is what happens when the brain has abnormal, uncontrolled electrical activity leading to a sudden change in a person's behavior. (Technically, a seizure can occur without any obvious change in behavior and even without the person being aware of it, but we will leave that for later.) So, you should think of a seizure as a single event. On the other hand, the term *epilepsy* is used to describe a condition in which a person has a tendency for recurrent seizures. Thus, rather than being a single event, epilepsy generally refers to a chronic condition. This definition means that a person who has had only one seizure does not have epilepsy. In fact, even two or three seizures might not mean a person has epilepsy, as long as the reason for the seizures can be fixed and there is no "tendency" or high likelihood for recurrences.

What Goes On in the Brain During a Seizure?

To understand what is going on in the brain during a seizure, you need to have a general idea of the brain structure. Everyone knows that the brain is a mass of gelatinous material that sits inside the skull and is responsible for our ability to think, speak, move our body, and sense the world, to name just a few of its amazing functions. Exactly how does the brain do these things? Neuroscientists have been working on this question for a long time now, and we are only beginning to get an idea of exactly how the brain accomplishes these tasks. However, we do know that one main cell type in the brain—the neuron—is a key player in brain function Figure 1.1. There are about 10 billion neurons in the human brain, and each neuron makes numerous connections with other neurons, forming an incredibly complex and intricate network. Some scientists have estimated that each neuron makes an average of 100,000 connections with other neurons, which means that the brain's neuronal network has a total of 1,000 trillion connections! Nature designed neurons to accomplish one main task—to communicate with one another by generating electrical impulses that can travel along the length of the cell and create a signal that influences the ability of other neurons to generate electrical impulses. Thus, neurons are miniature signaling devices that can detect incoming electrical impulses and, depending on the circumstances, relay the information to other cells in the form of electrical signals.

If it were possible to "listen" to the firing of electrical impulses by a large group of neurons during normal brain activity (for example, what your brain is doing right now as you read these words), you would hear many neurons firing away, but the overall sound would not make much sense. That is, the overall signaling occurring in the brain is so complex that the sum total of the firing by a large number of neurons would sound like chaotic noise. This chaotic, seemingly random activity is actually similar to what you can see with an electroencephalograph (EEG; a device

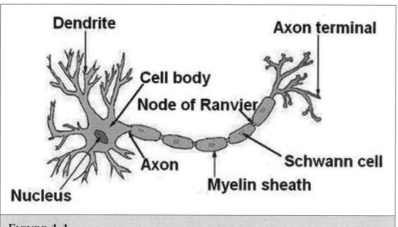

FIGURE 1.1

A typical neuron and its parts. The dendrite connects the neuron with other cells.

that measures the overall electrical activity of neurons) during normal brain function in a conscious person.

Now, here is the *key concept* in understanding what is going on in the brain when a person is having a seizure. During a seizure, large groups of neurons are out of control, they fire excessively, and they synchronize their firing with one another. Thus, if you were listening in on a group of neurons involved in a seizure, you would hear large-voltage, high-speed bursts of activity coming from many neurons at the same time—this is dramatically different from the relatively quiet and seemingly random background noise that you would hear normally.

A good way to visualize what is happening during a seizure is to imagine standing at the entrance of a large, busy restaurant and listening to the sounds of all the people talking at once. There are presumably meaningful conversations taking place at each table—whether it is the couple at a table for two or a large party of ten or twelve. However, the sound from where you are standing is just chaotic noise. If you think of each person in the restaurant as a neuron, you are hearing what the brain normally "sounds" like during normal activity. Now, imagine that suddenly a line of waiters and waitresses emerges from the kitchen. At the head of the line is a waiter carrying a birthday cake, and they are headed toward a table in the distance that is obviously the scene of a birthday celebration. As soon as the birthday cake comes into sight, the raucous group at the table begins singing "Happy Birthday" very loudly. Their loud singing represents the high-amplitude, super-synchronized activity that occurs in a group of neurons during a seizure. And you, standing at the doorway some distance from the singing, can detect this "abnormal" synchronized activity in much the same way that an EEG can detect seizure activity in the brain.

Believe it or not, this is really a fairly accurate analogy of what is going on in the brain during a seizure. As you will learn next, there are a variety of different seizure types, with the main distinguishing feature being whether the seizure activity stays restricted to just one part of the brain, or whether the seizure involves the entire brain. When a seizure stays restricted to one part of the brain, it is just like the song being sung by only the people at the birthday table. However, sometimes a seizure "focus" can spread to other regions of the brain, to the point at which the entire brain is undergoing a seizure—a so-called "generalized" seizure. This is analogous to people at neighboring tables joining in and singing the birthday song, to the point where every person in the restaurant is singing (loudly and synchronized!).

MORE ON THE DIFFERENT TYPES OF SEIZURES

As previously mentioned, a variety of seizure types exist, depending on where the abnormal neuronal activity is occurring. In fact, an internationally recognized seizure classification system is used by epilepsy doctors to try to make the most accurate diagnosis of a patient's problem and to provide a guide to the best therapy.

The basic classification system is shown in Table 1.1 and will explain each group in some detail.

Focal Seizures

Note that the first main category is "focal seizures." Focal seizures come from a discrete *focus* in the brain. That is, the abnormal firing of neurons start and stay restricted to one brain region.

TABLE 1.1
Classification of Seizures

I. Focal (or Partial) Seizures
    A.   Simple
       ▶ Motor
       ▶ Sensory
       ▶ Psychic
    B.   Complex
       ▶ Temporal lobe seizures
       ▶ Frontal lobe seizures

II. Generalized Seizures
    A.   Absence (petit mal)
    B.   Tonic–clonic (grand mal)
    C.   Atonic
    D.   Myoclonic

III. Focal (or Partial) Seizures with Secondary Generalization

---

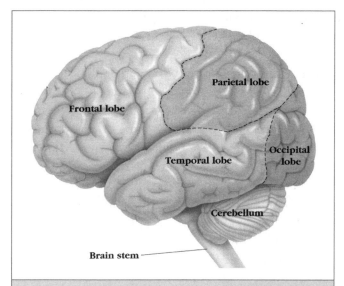

FIGURE 1.2
The human brain with the different lobes. This is a view of the left hemisphere.

To confuse matters somewhat, the classification system uses the term "partial" synonymously with "focal." Many people misinterpret the term "partial" to mean that a seizure is partial or incomplete– but that is not the case. Just substitute the word "focal" every time you hear "partial."

To understand the different types of focal seizures, you need to have a general appreciation for how the brain is organized. You can see in Figure 1.2 that each half of the brain is composed of four major regions or "lobes," and, as a general rule, each one of these lobes has a distinctive set of functions. The *occipital lobe* at the back of the brain analyzes the signals coming from the eye and enables us to see. The *parietal lobe*, just in front of the occipital lobe, interprets information coming from sensory receptors throughout the body—it is responsible for our ability to feel skin sensations, including things like light touch, temperature, pain, and the position of our limbs. The *temporal lobe* sits below the parietal lobe and allows us to form memories, experience emotions and, along with the frontal lobe, use language. (Actually, language typically resides on one side of the brain or the other; in the majority of people this on the left half of the brain.) Finally, the frontal lobe, at the front of the brain, is responsible for many of the higher-level functions that are the most distinctive of human traits such as judgment, planning, personality, planning, and abstract reasoning. Also, a very important function of the *frontal lobe* (coming from the back-most part right next to the border with the parietal lobe) is the control of motor movements.

Now, back to the question of the various types of focal seizures. Since different parts of the brain do different things, the nature of the seizure, or the behavior you might observe in a person during a seizure, will depend on which part of the brain is undergoing seizure activity. Suppose, for example, we could create a seizure focus precisely in the part of the frontal lobe that is responsible for motor movement. Since the seizure focus creates uncontrolled activity in a group of neurons, the seizure that the person experiences may be uncontrolled shaking movements of the arm, the leg, the face, or a combination of these, depending on the extent of the region involved. This would not cause any abnormality of awareness or consciousness in the person, so we classify the seizure as being simple (rather than complex) because the nature of the abnormal behavior is relatively simple. In the classification system shown in Table 1.1, the seizure we just created would be called a *simple focal (or partial) motor seizure.*

If we created a seizure focus slightly farther back in the brain—in the parietal lobe—the person might experience odd sensations, since the parietal lobe is responsible for (among other things) detecting sensations in the skin. In this case, an outside observer might not detect anything obviously wrong (for example, abnormal movements or behavior). Again, this type of seizure activity would not cause any abnormality of awareness or consciousness, so we classify the seizure as a *simple focal (or partial) sensory seizure.*

What happens when the seizure focus is located in the temporal or frontal lobe? Now things get a bit more complicated, because most functions of these two parts of the brain are more complex than the regions just described (refer to Figure 1.1). For example, let's place the seizure focus in the left temporal lobe. In this case, the seizure activity would disrupt the normal function of the brain dealing with memory, emotions, and possibly language. Try to imagine what you would feel like if you suddenly were unable to remember anything (such as recognizing the faces of people around you), you became anxious (because your emotions were difficult to control), and you were unable to speak or understand the words other people were saying. This interruption of your normal thinking would cause you to have an abnormal level of consciousness. To an outside observer, you might appear confused (e.g., with a dazed, "far off" look), perhaps afraid, and unable to communicate with others. For reasons we don't fully understand, seizures of this type can also cause repetitive, automatic-like behaviors, such as lip smacking or picking movements of the hands, which are called *automatisms.* As you can see, this type of focal seizure has much more complex behaviors associated with it, compared with the simple motor seizure and simple sensory seizure described earlier. It is therefore classified as a *complex focal (or partial) seizure.*

A somewhat similar situation occurs when the seizure originates in the frontal lobe. Again, the abnormal neuronal activity would disrupt functions of the brain such as judgment and abstract reasoning, so you can see how the person with a frontal lobe seizure might have an interruption of his normal consciousness. We would therefore classify this seizure as being a complex focal (or partial) seizure emanating from frontal lobe onset, as opposed to onset from the temporal lobe.

Not surprisingly, focal seizures can cross the boundaries of the various lobes of the brain or involve multiple functions. So, for example, a focal seizure of the frontal lobe might not only cause a change in a person's consciousness, but it could also cause abnormal motor movements due to the involvement of the region of the frontal lobe responsible for the control of movement.

We want to review one last point before moving on to the other main categories of seizures. You may have noticed that we skipped over a simple focal seizure categorized as "psychic." This generally refers to a seizure that is coming from the temporal lobe or frontal lobe and causes an odd awareness that something is not quite right, such as a feeling of rushed thoughts, déjà vu (feeling as though you have already experienced what is happening around you), sudden emotions (e.g., fear), or sensing unusual odors or sounds. These seizures are similar to what may be experienced during complex focal seizures, but no impairment of consciousness occurs. That is, the person is awake and aware of what is going on, and can describe it to others. Since consciousness is not impaired, this is classified as a *simple focal (or partial) psychic seizure*. Also, these particular experiences are usually what is meant when a person says he is having an aura. An aura can occur as a stand-alone event, but it often progresses into a complex focal seizure. People with epilepsy quickly learn that an *aura* is a warning sign that a larger seizure may be coming. (In fact, the word "aura" comes from the Greek word meaning "breeze," as if the breeze is a signal that a storm may soon follow.)

Generalized Seizures

Generalized seizures are, not surprisingly, quite different from focal seizures, because the abnormal neuronal firing seems to occur in most of the brain all at once. Purists might say that a seizure cannot possibly start precisely all over the brain at exactly the same time—it must start somewhere! And they are probably right. However, in practical terms, a generalized seizure takes over the brain so quickly that it is impossible (using current methods) to detect where the first electrical discharge begins.

Absence (also called *petit mal*) seizures are a distinctive type of seizure in which a sudden abnormality occurs in the circuitry that connects the surface of the brain with a deeper structure called the *thalamus*. Interestingly, these are the same pathways that enable us to transition from being awake and being asleep, and there are some parallels between the behavior of a person having an absence seizure and being asleep. During the seizure, which usually starts abruptly and without warning, the person just goes blank for a few seconds. There may be a small amount of facial movements, such as fluttering of the eyelids or movements of the mouth, but the patient otherwise maintains his posture or position, and the seizure stops as abruptly as it began. People are usually able to maintain their posture during the seizure—for example, they can remain standing. These seizures tend to occur in children, and the EEG shows a very characteristic wave pattern that is known as "3-per-second spike-and-wave" that emanates from the so-called *thalamo-cortical* circuitry.

Probably the most commonly recognized seizure type is the tonic–clonic (or *grand mal*) seizure. The seizure activity seems to instantaneously spread over both sides of the brain, leading to a loss of consciousness. Since the part of the brain controlling motor movement is affected on both sides of the brain, the person usually has stiffening of the arms and legs on both sides of the body, and this causes him to fall if standing up. The stiffening is referred to as the *tonic phase*. Depending on when the seizure begins during the breathing cycle, the sudden contraction of the muscles of the diaphragm and the voice box may cause the person to let out a very unusual cry. After a short while, the constant stiffening is replaced by cycles of stiffening and relaxation of the muscles, which leads to shaking movements (the *clonic phase*). Finally, once the seizure passes, the person becomes limp and remains unconscious until the brain recovers sufficiently to allow the person to wake up again. The duration of tonic–clonic seizures can vary a great deal, but the tonic and clonic phases usually last about a minute or two, and it usually takes at least 15 to 30 minutes (and often longer) for a person to begin to return to normal.

A more unusual generalized seizure is an *atonic seizure.* "Atonic" refers to a loss of tone, so you can imagine what happens when a seizure of this type suddenly occurs while a person is upright. The person abruptly becomes limp and collapses to the ground. Many individuals with this form of seizure must wear a protective helmet to prevent serious head injury from falling. It might be a bit difficult to understand how hyperexcitable, super-synchronized neurons could lead to a *loss* of tone rather than increased tone. However, researchers have learned that the overall output of certain networks of activated neurons can be inhibitory rather than excitatory; it is thought that this is the basis for atonic seizures.

Myoclonic seizures refer to extremely brief, jerking movements. The movements are the same as the very sudden movement that can occur when a normal person is falling asleep in a classroom, for example. A myoclonic seizure can be a single jerking movement lasting a fraction of a second, or repetitive jerking movements lasting seconds or minutes (and rarely longer). These are frequently seen in people who have other types of generalized seizures.

Focal (or Partial) Seizures with Secondary Generalization

If you have a good idea of what is happening in a focal seizure versus what is happening in a generalized seizure, then this last main category of seizures, called *focal (or partial) seizures with secondary generalization*, should not be too difficult to understand. Imagine a focal seizure beginning in the part of the frontal lobe controlling motor movements. As we discussed before, this would lead to shaking movements of the arm, leg, or face. But now imagine that the overall state of the brain is such that the brain tissue surrounding the seizure focus is relatively susceptible to abnormal excitation and, under certain conditions, can be "recruited" to join in to the seizure focus. In this case, the seizure focus will begin to grow and spread, and it can rather quickly take over the entire brain. Thus, the person who was initially having shaking movements in one part of the body will become unconscious (and fall to the ground if upright) and have the other manifestations of a generalized seizure. It is important to try to discriminate between a pure, generalized seizure and a focal seizure with secondary generalization, because the causes of these two types of seizures can be quite different.

EPILEPTIC SYNDROMES

In addition to classifying seizures, experts in the field have developed a separate classification system for the different epilepsies or epileptic syndromes. Classifying epilepsy by seizure type alone creates problems when an individual has more than one seizure type. In addition, it leaves out other critical information that may be important in understanding each individual's condition. When doctors classify an individual as having a specific epilepsy syndrome, they take into account a number of characteristics including seizure type, EEG recordings, age of onset of the seizures, family history, precipitating features, and accompanying neurologic symptoms or problems. Making a diagnosis of a specific epileptic syndrome often allows the physician to provide more accurate information about the expected response to treatment and better counseling regarding the possibility that the epilepsy may be inherited. An understanding of the epilepsy syndrome may also affect what treatment the doctor chooses for the seizures.

Table 1.2 provides a simple outline for the classification scheme for the epilepsies and epileptic syndromes. It is based on an international classification scheme that is much more complex and beyond the focus of this discussion. Just as with the classification of seizures, the classification of the epileptic syndromes is divided into those with focal-onset seizures (*localization-related* or *focal epilepsies*) or generalized seizures (the *generalized epilepsies*). Within both the localized and generalized groups are additional subdivisions into *idiopathic* (unknown cause, often determined to be genetic), *symptomatic* (identified cause), and *cryptogenic* (hidden cause).

Under the heading of localization-related epilepsies, most of the syndromes are defined by where in the brain the seizures originate, such as in the temporal, frontal, parietal, or occipital lobes. For example, in frontal lobe epilepsy, there are examples of idiopathic, symptomatic, and cryptogenic subtypes. An example of an idiopathic frontal lobe epilepsy is the syndrome of *autosomal dominant nocturnal frontal lobe epilepsy*. This syndrome initially had no identified cause but was recognized to occur in families. Eventually, it led to the identification of a specific gene for a particular chemical receptor that caused the syndrome. In many cases, the use of the term *idiopathic* implies that the cause of the epilepsy is thought to be genetic. Frontal lobe epilepsy may also arise from a structural lesion in the frontal lobe that can be seen on magnetic resonance imaging (MRI). When we are able to identify an abnormality in the frontal lobe that is the cause of the seizures (such as a tumor or blood vessel abnormality), the syndrome is classified as *symptomatic frontal lobe epilepsy*. Similarly, many individuals diagnosed with frontal lobe epilepsy have no identified cause (even after exhaustive testing); they are labeled as having *cryptogenic epilepsy*. Here, the doctors believe that a scar or brain abnormality is present, but it is just too small to discover with our present tools.

The most common example of a symptomatic localization-related epilepsy occurs in *temporal lobe epilepsy*. The temporal lobe, an area of the brain that sits on each side of the head just above the ear, is the most common site for the onset of epileptic seizures. Individuals with temporal lobe epilepsy frequently have a history of brain insult in infancy, such as a prolonged fever-related seizure (complex febrile seizure) or brain infection (bacterial meningitis). Many years later, complex partial seizures develop that are often difficult to control with medicines. The EEG shows abnormal epileptiform or spike activity over one or both temporal lobes. The MRI, particularly when special images are done through the temporal lobe, reveals scaring or shrinkage of the hippocampus. The *hippocampus* is a structure deep within the temporal lobe that is primarily involved in memory but, for unclear reasons, is also very likely to give rise to seizures. **Many patients with temporal lobe epilepsy are not controlled with antiepileptic drug treatment.** These individuals with uncontrolled *mesial temporal lobe epilepsy* are often treated with surgery to take out the scarred hippocampus, and this surgery has an excellent chance of stopping the seizures.

The second category of epilepsy syndromes, the generalized epileptic syndromes, centers on individuals with predominantly generalized seizures and includes many of the most common epileptic syndromes such as *juvenile myoclonic epilepsy*, *childhood absence epilepsy*, *infantile spasms*, and *Lennox-Gastaut syndrome*. All these syndromes will be discussed in subsequent chapters.

A few uncommon epileptic syndromes appear to have features of both generalized and localization-related seizures and are classified in a third and separate category in Table 1.2. An example of this type is the *Landau-Kleffner syndrome* (LKS), which is also called acquired *epileptic aphasia*. LKS is a syndrome characterized by two major symptoms: the development of aphasia or language impairment and a profoundly abnormal EEG with epileptiform activity occurring over the temporal regions and/or in a generalized distribution. It usually has its onset between the ages of 3 and 8 years. Seizures do occur, but are much less of a problem than the cognitive and language impairments.

The fourth category of epileptic syndromes is called *special syndromes*. These are often syndromes that are clearly defined but are so different that they do not fit comfortably into any of the other three categories. Two examples include *febrile seizures* and *reflex epilepsy*. **A febrile seizure is a specific syndrome that involves generalized seizures occurring with a fever.** Not all experts consider this a true form of epilepsy, but it does appear in the international classification. Febrile seizures occur in 3% to 4% of children, usually between the ages of 6 months to 5 years of age, with the peak being at approximately 18 months of age. Children with febrile seizures are usually not treated because the seizures occur infrequently and the medicines are of

---

TABLE **1.2**

Simplified Classification of Epilepsies and Epileptic Syndromes

I.   Localization-related (involves one or more distinct areas of the brain)

II. Generalized (involves both sides of the brain at the same time)

III. Undetermined whether localized or generalized

IV. Special syndromes

questionable effectiveness. Most children simply outgrow the tendency to have seizures with fever and never have problems with seizures again. However, approximately 5% of children with febrile seizures will develop focal or localization-related epilepsy later in life, particularly if the febrile seizures were very long or had other complicated features. Reflex epilepsy is an uncommon but fascinating group of disorders that is also considered under the heading of special syndromes. Reflex epilepsy is the name given to seizures that are triggered by sensitivity to sensory stimulation in the environment. The most common form is *photosensitive epilepsy*, in which seizures are precipitated by exposure to intense or fluctuating levels of light such as those given off by a strobe light. The condition usually begins in childhood and is usually outgrown by adulthood. Other rare triggers for reflex epilepsy include certain sounds, reading, immersion in hot water, and even eating.

CAUSES OF EPILEPSY

When a person is told that she has epilepsy, many questions immediately come to mind. Usually the first question is "Why me?" Understandably, you want to know what is causing your seizure disorder. Despite the development of sensitive tests such as MRI, doctors still are unable to identify the cause of epilepsy in about half of individuals with the new onset of epilepsy. When doctors are able to identify a cause for epilepsy, the likely cause varies depending on the age when seizures begin. Newborn infants very frequently have seizures due to problems surrounding their birth; this will be discussed in a later chapter (Chapter 7). In young children, common causes of epilepsy include abnormalities in the brain present at birth and infections in the central nervous system. These nervous system infections include meningitis (an infection of the covering of the brain and spinal cord) or encephalitis (an infection of the brain itself). When epilepsy begins in a school-age child, genetics often plays a prominent role. The specific genetic pattern of inheritance is often complex, but it is clear that many seizure disorders, particularly those discussed under generalized epileptic seizures (see Table 1.2) are due to a genetic predisposition. In adolescents and young adults, head trauma (particularly if associated with loss of consciousness or accompanied by bleeding in or around the brain) often leads to the development of epilepsy. When adults develop epilepsy, the first concern usually is "Do I have a brain tumor?" Although brain tumors of all sorts are a possible cause of epilepsy throughout adulthood, they represent only a small percentage of all cases of new-onset epilepsy. A much more common cause of epilepsy is stroke. A *stroke* is an injury to the brain that occurs when the blood supply to an area of the brain is cut off. Strokes happen much more frequently in the elderly and, as a result, epilepsy is surprisingly common in older individuals. Epilepsy is widely thought to be a disorder of childhood, but it is common at any age, and the largest number of new-onset cases of epilepsy is actually in people over the age of 65.

FACTORS THAT MAY PROVOKE SEIZURES

Even in people without epilepsy, seizures can be provoked if enough biologic stresses are present. In fact about 10% of people will have a seizure sometime in their life, but only about 1% will go on to have epilepsy (meaning recurrent unprovoked seizures). Some have seizures with a high fever as an infant or child (febrile seizures discussed earlier); others will have a seizure due to the effect of a medical illness (kidney failure) or drugs (both street drugs or prescription drugs). Everybody has a certain *threshold* or propensity to have seizures. The difference in an individual with epilepsy is that the threshold (or "hurdle") is lower, and it is easier to "get over" the threshold and go on to have a seizure. The use of antiepileptic drugs helps raise that seizure threshold, making it less likely a seizure will occur.

However, many things that happen in your day-to-day life may lower that seizure threshold and, as a result, make having a seizure more likely. The two most common lifestyle factors that provoke seizures are sleep-deprivation and alcohol. Sleep deprivation can be due to staying up all night, one night (such as when trying to finish a school or work project) or can be due to being short on sleep over several days or weeks due to work or social demands. The bottom line is that getting adequate rest is very important for anyone with a seizure disorder. Alcoholic beverages are also a very common cause of breakthrough seizures. Having several alcoholic drinks very clearly lowers your seizure threshold and makes seizures more likely. It is less clear whether a single alcoholic drink helps bring on seizures, but avoiding alcohol altogether is commonly recommended for anyone with epilepsy. Other stresses that may push you toward having seizures are listed in Table 1.3.

In Table 1.3, drugs, both recreational and medical, are identified to lower the seizure threshold. Of the recreational or street drugs, stimulants (such as cocaine) and hallucinogens (PCP) seem

---

TABLE 1.3
Factors That Lower Seizure Threshold

Common:	Occasional:
Sleep deprivation	Hyperventilation
Alcohol	Flashing lights
Infection (fever)	Stress (physical, emotional)
Recreational drugs (cocaine, stimulants)	Medications (sedating antihistamines, some antibiotics)
Menstruation	

to be the drugs that most commonly cause seizures. Several over-the-counter (OTC) or prescription medicines can also bring on seizures. Sedating antihistamines (which are found in many multisymptom cold or allergy remedies) are the OTC medicines that seem to most commonly precipitate breakthrough seizures. A few prescribed medications (such as the antibiotic ciprofloxacin [Cipro]) also are reported to increase the risk of seizures.

Many people with epilepsy attempt to identify factors in their daily life that seem to bring on seizures. Diet is often examined as a possible cause, but most evidence suggests that diet (specific foods or missed meals) is rarely a significant contributor to seizure risk. Many women identify an increase in seizures with their menstrual cycle, and this is supported in the scientific literature. An increase in seizures is commonly seen just at the onset of menstrual flow or during midcycle (at the time of ovulation).

THE RISKS OR DANGERS ASSOCIATED WITH HAVING SEIZURES

Do Seizures Cause Brain Injury?

Up until about 10 years ago the answer to this question was easy and simple: No, a single isolated seizures, whether partial or generalized, does not cause injury to brain cells. Only if the seizure activity was prolonged (>30 minutes) did doctors begin to worry about the possibility of permanent brain injury due to seizure activity. However, over the last 10 years, evidence has accumulated in animal studies (as well as some evidence in human studies) that even recurrent isolated seizures can lead to further brain injury. In real life, though, the majority of people with epilepsy, even after years of active problems with seizures, still have no evidence of additional brain injury or brain function impairment. So, while complete seizure control is obviously everyone's goal, recurrent seizure activity is rarely identified to cause additional injury to the brain.

Risks of Injury During a Seizure

A major concern to many people with epilepsy is the possibility of injury during a seizure. During a tonic–clonic seizure, an intense and unnatural muscle contraction occurs beyond what anyone can carry out voluntarily. This results in the muscle soreness that frequently is noted in the days after a convulsive seizure. Often the tongue may be bitten as the jaw muscles clamp down. This can be extremely painful, but unfortunately cannot be prevented because the contraction usually occurs too quickly for any intervention. The intense muscle contraction can also sometimes result in shoulder dislocations or compression fractures of the spine. Shoulder dislocations are painful but can be *reduced* or put back in place in the emergency department. A *compression fracture* of the spine is probably more common and occurs when the muscles surrounding the vertebrae in your spine contract so strongly that they compress or partially collapse one of the bones that makes up your spinal column. This does not lead to injury to the spinal cord, but results in significant pain over the area of the compression.

With tonic–clonic seizures, abrupt loss of consciousness *usually occurs*, so that falls from the standing position are common. Individuals with active seizure problems are counseled to avoid dangerous activities (working at heights, operating large machinery, swimming alone) in which that they would be at a markedly increased risk if they suffered a seizure. In a fall from a standing position, any number of injuries can occur: head trauma, broken bones, cuts, and bruises. Significant head trauma is the most worrisome for fear of concussions, brain contusions, and bleeding inside the skull. This is why that some people with uncontrolled epilepsy, particularly with frequent tonic, atonic, or tonic–clonic seizures, may be required to wear a helmet to avoid serious brain injury.

FREQUENTLY ASKED QUESTIONS

Q My doctor says he doesn't know the cause of my seizures, so why do I have them?

A The two terms doctors use to describe your epilepsy, if there is no evident cause, are *cryptogenic* or *idiopathic*. Cryptogenic comes from the Greek words meaning "obscure or unknown origin." Idiopathic comes from the Greek words meaning "one's own private suffering." In either case, these terms are a fancy way of saying that the cause of your epilepsy remains unknown to the doctor. In most cases of cryptogenic epilepsy, it is likely that a small brain abnormality is present that is too small to be discovered by any of our tests. This small area of abnormality cannot be seen on the MRI, but still is able to cause the abnormal electrical activity that leads to your seizure. When doctors use the term idiopathic epilepsy, it has come to imply that the cause is likely to be genetic. Even in idiopathic epilepsy, it is common not to have a clear family history, but the clinical suspicion focuses on an inherited trait that may have predisposed you to developing epilepsy.

Q I'm told my seizures are coming from a scar on my brain that occurred during an auto accident 10 years ago. Why did it take so long for my seizures to show up?

A To have a delay of months or even years after a brain injury before the development of epilepsy is very common. Exactly what is going on in the brain during this interval is unknown. Scientists continue to explore the changes that are happening to the brain cells during this time, but the answer as to why epilepsy develops after this delay is not completely known. The hope is that with better understanding of this process, doctors may be able to intervene during the "lull in the action" and prevent the subsequent development of epilepsy. Unfortunately, no medicine or treatment has been identified that can interrupt this process in humans.

Q How can I tell what type of seizures I have?

A Your doctor combines the information from your history (age of onset, description of your seizure behavior, risk factors for epilepsy) and medical tests (EEG, MRI) to determine the type of seizures that you have. If your seizures begin before the age of 15, about half will be focal (or partial) in onset and half will be generalized in onset. The presence of an abnormality on your MRI or focal epilepsy–type changes on your EEG, would make the diagnosis of a focal or partial epilepsy likely. If the EEG showed a generalized pattern, a generalized epilepsy would likely be the diagnosis. This information is then combined with the clinical history, including a description of the seizures themselves, to make the diagnosis or determination. The doctor uses your description of your seizures and combines it with what observers say about your seizures to get as clear a picture as possible about the type of seizures that you are experiencing. However, sometimes the tests are all normal, and the description of the seizure is not conclusive enough to allow a diagnosis of a specific seizure type. In older individuals, say over 30 or 35 year old, it is much easier. Almost everybody presenting with new-onset seizures in this age group will have partial epilepsy. The doctor then uses the description of the seizures to determine whether you are having simple partial seizures, complex partial seizures, or secondarily generalized tonic–clonic seizures (see Table 1.2).

Q Can I die from having a seizure?

A The biggest danger from a seizure comes from what the individual is doing when a seizure occurs. Obviously, if you are driving a car, there is a real risk of serious injury to yourself and others. So lifestyle restrictions (such as not driving, not swimming alone, not working at heights) are the first steps to assuring the safety of someone with uncontrolled seizures. As discussed in this chapter, there are also risks from falls during the seizure or from confusion after the seizure. However, the seizure itself, although often terrifying to observe, is not immediately life threatening. Rarely, individuals with epilepsy can suffer an unexpected sudden death. These episodes usually are unwitnessed and occur more commonly in poorly controlled epilepsy. The exact cause or causes remain unknown. Thankfully, *sudden unexpected death in epilepsy* (often abbreviated SUDEP) is extremely rare.

Q When should I call for emergency help?

A When someone witnesses a convulsive or tonic–clonic seizure for the first time, emergency help will almost always be summoned due to the frightening nature of the seizure and the fear that the person is dying or seriously ill. However, in someone with an established diagnosis of epilepsy, emergency help does not need to be summoned for each seizure. Proper "seizure first-aid" should be carried out (see Appendix) and the person observed until achieving a normal degree of alertness. However, there are situations in which it is appropriate to summon emergency help, even in someone who has an established diagnosis of epilepsy. There are three main situations in which summoning emergency assistance is appropriate:

▶ If the seizure duration (active motor jerking) lasts more than 5 minutes (as timed by a clock).

▶ If the person has a second seizure before regaining a normal degree of alertness.

▶ If the person has injured himself significantly during the seizure (such as a head injury due to a fall).

These are general guidelines and are not meant to replace your doctor's advice and instructions. Please discuss and consult with your physician on the details of your particular form of epilepsy.

My Notes

_____

_____

_____

_____

_____

_____

_____

2

DIAGNOSIS OF SEIZURES AND EPILEPSY

Clinical and Laboratory Tests

Key Points

▶ Approximately 90% of the new-onset cases in adults have partial ("part" of the brain is involved with seizure onset) epilepsy.

▶ With the occurrence of a first seizure or a recurrence of a first seizure, it is important to seek an explanation or a cause.

▶ The electroencephalogram (EEG) is the only test that can prove that somebody has epilepsy.

▶ Patients with seizure disorders, even medically intractable epilepsy, may have repetitive "normal" EEG studies.

▶ Video-EEG monitoring is predominantly used by most physicians for diagnostic classification.

▶ MRI is the best imaging technique we have to find the cause of seizures.

▶ It is not uncommon for patients with psychogenic events to have many normal EEG recordings.

AS WE LEARNED IN CHAPTER 1, epilepsy is a chronic medical condition characterized by recurrent and unprovoked seizures. It is one of the most common neurologic disorders. The lifetime risk of developing epilepsy is almost 4%. Approximately 90% of the new-onset cases in adults have partial ("part" of the brain is involved with seizure onset) epilepsy. Nearly 70% of partial seizures are associated with temporal lobe epilepsy; that is, seizures arising from the temporal lobe in the brain.

As we will see, the abnormal behavior or symptoms associated with seizures and the area of the brain involved with the seizure onset are used to understand and classify the seizure activity (Tables 2.1 and 2.2). As explained in Chapter 1, the generalized seizures (involving both the right and left side of the brain at onset) include *tonic–clonic* (grand mal or convulsions), *absence* (petit mal), *myoclonic*, *atonic* (drop attacks), and *tonic* (increased tone in the arms and legs). Partial seizures include *complex partial* (behavioral arrest and staring), *simple partial* (patient remains awake), or *secondarily generalized tonic-clonic* (part of the brain initiates a tonic–clonic seizure). It is important to remember that the majority of convulsions (generalized tonic–clonic seizures) are partial in onset with secondary generalization (see Table 1.1). The distinction between complex and simple partial seizures depends on the presence of impairment in consciousness during the seizure, and making this distinction can be challenging.

ESTABLISHING A DIAGNOSIS OF SEIZURES AND EPILEPSY

With the occurrence of a first seizure or a recurrence of a first seizure, it is important to seek an explanation or a cause. A medical doctor (MD) or physician should be consulted. As in any other field of medicine, there are specialists who are trained in the diagnosis and treatment of seizures. For those 18 years and older, a neurologist will be the most appropriate physician; for children, a pediatric neurologist should be consulted. Some neurologists specialize in epilepsy (epileptologist), and those may be particularly appropriate when seizures are difficult to control or when other treatments are needed.

Several steps are taken in the neurologic consultation and investigation of patients with seizures or epilepsy. These steps are:

1. Clinical evaluation
2. Laboratory testing
3. Neurophysiologic testing

TABLE **2.1**
Differential Diagnoses in Patients with Possible Epilepsy

1.   The physiologic causes of these spells include:
   a.   Cardiac syncope
   b.   Vasodepressor syncope
   c.   Simple faint
   d.   Migraine
   e.   Movement disorder
   f.   Hyperventilation
   g.   Cerebrovascular disease
   h.   Autonomic disorder
   i.   Drug toxicity
   j.   Vertigo and dizziness
   k.   Sleep disorders
2.   The psychological causes include:
   a.   Panic attacks
   b.   Mood disorder
   c.   Behavioral events (pseudoseizures)
   d.   Psychotic episodes
   e.   Anxiety disorder

Differential diagnoses
Nonepileptic disorders may present a diagnostic challenge in the individual with epilepsy. Many individuals with nonepileptic paroxysmal disorders do not have a determined *etiology* or cause for their spells, despite an extensive evaluation. Most of these patients have either behavioral events (*pseudoseizures*) or indeterminate spells.

4.   Neuroimaging
5.   Other special tests

Clinical Evaluation

The clinical evaluation takes place when a patient walks into the neurologist's office or when the neurologist sees the patient in the hospital. The visit is first directed at establishing the details of the seizure and the patient's medical history. This is one of the most important aspects of the evaluation. The physician will try to establish whether the seizure was indeed a seizure, or if it was something that looked like a seizure but may be something else (Table 2.1).

This part of the evaluation is called the *differential diagnosis*, and it is very important since a number of conditions can look like epileptic seizures.

Let's suppose that the initial interview suggests a seizure. The physician will try to establish whether the seizure's features are consistent with the typical expected manifestations. For example, was there an aura? Did the patient lose consciousness? Did any motor activity occur? Were vision changes experienced? Was the tongue bitten? Because the patient may have lost consciousness during the seizure, it is a good idea to have along someone else who witnessed the event, or at least be available to answer the doctor's questions.

Once the patient's history, including any other medical issues in addition to the seizure event, has been obtained, the physician performs a physical and neurologic examination. The physical examination may uncover clues to the cause of the seizure. For example, certain skin lesions are associated with a brain disorder called *tuberous sclerosis*, which can present with epilepsy (see Chapter 7). Other physical changes the neurologist will look for may include weakness or sensory changes in one part of the body, visual field loss, or other symptoms. Once the history and physical examination have been completed, the neurologist will establish an impression and design a plan of action.

General Laboratory Testing

In the context of a first seizure, it is often necessary to run some routine tests that may explain the cause of the seizure. A number of changes in the normal blood composition can induce a seizure. The most common changes are reductions in sodium (salt) or glucose (sugar). The presence of drugs, both legal and illegal, may be the cause of a seizure. Some antipsychotics, asthma medications, stimulants, and antidepressants can cause seizures. Similarly, cocaine, heroine, and other illegal drugs can induce seizures. For that reason, a *drug screen* is often done the first time a seizure takes place in certain patients. An *electrocardiogram* (EKG) is also done to check for potential heart problems that may present like a seizure. For some patients with recurrent seizures associated with other conditions, specialized laboratory testing is done but these are much less commonly needed.

Neurophysiologic Studies

Routine Electroencephalography

The electroencephalogram (EEG) is the only test that can prove that somebody has epilepsy. The brain produces electrical activity that may be analyzed using an EEG machine. A routine EEG in the office or hospital is typically collected for 30 to 60 minutes by the application of metal electrodes placed on the scalp with a conducting paste (Figure 2.1). The electrodes are attached to wires that connect to the input box of the EEG machine. The EEG machine displays the electrical activity on a computer screen or paper (Figure 2.2). The outpatient scalp-recorded EEG predominantly observes *interictal* (brain activity between seizures) EEG changes, and may be altered by the presence of antiepileptic medications and other factors.

The human brain has fairly predictable electrical activity that varies with its location within the brain and whether the person being recorded is awake or asleep (Figure 2.3). In people with epilepsy, the EEG shows evidence of irritability, reported as either as spike or sharp wave. These abnormal waves are a hallmark of epilepsy, and they occur even when a person with epilepsy is not experiencing a seizure. Spikes and sharp waves may occur in one location, multiple locations, or throughout the entire brain at once (Figures 2.4 and 2.5). The type and localization of the epilepsy you have can sometimes be diagnosed when these discharges are recorded with an EEG. Spikes and sharp waves may be provoked by sleep, deep breathing (hyperventilation), or flashing lights (photic stimulation).

Although the EEG may tell your neurologist if you have epilepsy, it may not tell him what type of epilepsy you have. EEG studies are not always reliable indicators of the classification of

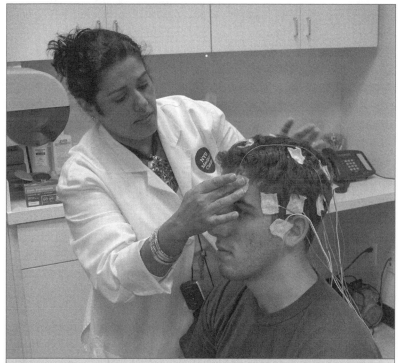

FIGURE 2.1
Patient being prepared with electrodes for an EEG scan.

seizure type. The routine EEG may be insensitive to (it may fail to identify) *epileptiform discharges*, which are abnormalities associated with an increased risk of seizure activity, or it may yield nonspecific findings. EEG alterations may rarely be identified in a patient with nonepileptic behavioral events. Patients with seizure disorders, even medically intractable epilepsy, may have repetitive "normal" EEG studies.

If a laboratory or office EEG does not detect an abnormality, the physician

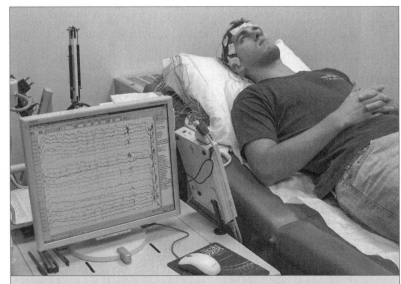

FIGURE 2.2
Patient undergoing EEG study in the office. Computer screen showing the collection of an EEG. The study usually takes one hour.

may order a *sleep-deprived EEG*, during which the patient is kept awake all night and an EEG is obtained while he is awake and then asleep. If the EEG is still inconclusive or unrevealing, your doctor may order an *outpatient ambulatory EEG*, or he may want to hospitalize you for *video-EEG monitoring*.

Ambulatory Electroencephalography

An ambulatory EEG uses basically the same technology as a regular in-office EEG, but instead of recording activity for 30 to 60 minutes, it records the patient's brain activity for days at a time. The patient carries a small pouch or device on his belt, while the electrodes are attached to his or her head (Figure 2.6). The ambulatory EEG device runs on batteries and has memory cards that can store EEG data for several days. Most ambulatory EEG studies are run for 24 to 72 hours. The advantage of ambulatory EEG is that it can record your EEG for one or more days, and it might detect abnormal discharges that are very infrequent. The other

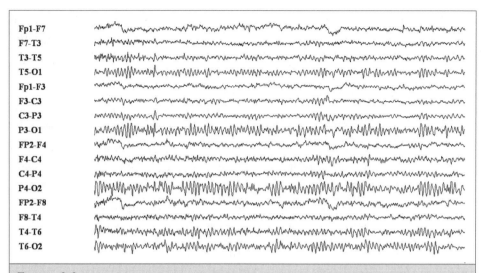

FIGURE 2.3

Normal, adult, awake EEG with normal alpha activity (T5-O1, P3-O1, P4-O2, T6-O2).

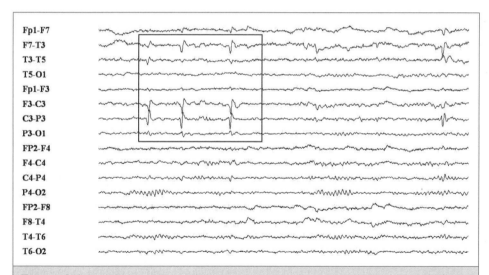

FIGURE 2.4

EEG showing focal spikes (interictal EEG) in a patient with left centro-temporal lobe epilepsy.

major advantage is that it may record actual seizures, which seldom can be recorded on the routine EEG (Figure 2.7). In those cases, the electrical activity can be analyzed, and sometimes an opinion can be formed regarding where in the brain seizures might be starting.

Video-Electroencephalographic Monitoring

If the routine EEG and/or the ambulatory EEG are negative, or do not provide a definite answer on the diagnosis, your doctor may refer you for video-EEG monitoring. This is typically done in the setting of a specialized epilepsy monitoring unit in a hospital. The technology is similar to a routine EEG or ambulatory EEG except that a video camera is running during the EEG recording (Figure 2.8). The main advantage of video-EEG is that the neurologist can observe seizures and correlate the EEG with the seizure behavior. Trained nurses or EEG technologists can also perform testing during the seizure. Because seizures may occur relatively infrequently in some people, antiepileptic medication can be reduced or stopped to induce seizures.

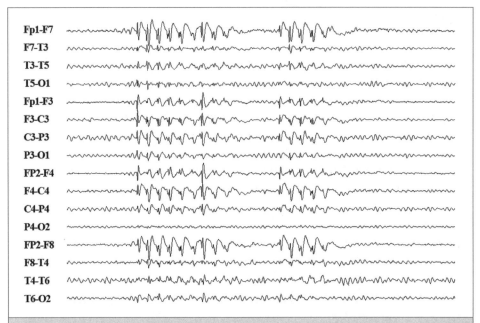

FIGURE 2.5
Generalized spike and wave abnormality (interictal EEG) in an awake patient with primary generalized epilepsy.

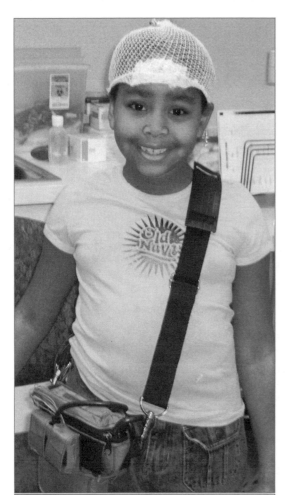

FIGURE 2.6
Young patient carrying an ambulatory EEG pack. EEG electrodes are connected to the head as with a routine EEG.

Additional body changes that can be evaluated during video-EEG monitoring include heart rhythm (using an electrocardiogram [EKG]), and changes in blood pressure, heart rate, and breathing. These assessments may be necessary in differentiating a seizure from other medical events, such as passing out from a drop in blood pressure. In addition, seizure-inducing maneuvers can also be done, such as sleep deprivation. People may be admitted to the hospital for a few days or up to a week, depending on how often their seizures occur and how many need to be studied. In some patients, video-EEG monitoring may be essential in the care and management of patient's seizure disorder.

Video-EEG monitoring is predominantly used by most physicians for diagnostic classification; that is, to determine epileptic from nonepileptic events, to classify the seizure type and syndrome, and sometimes to count the number of seizures and to evaluate whether a patient is a good candidate for epilepsy surgery (see Chapter 5). The high value of video-EEG monitoring in children and adult patients with recurrent and unprovoked spells has been confirmed by many studies and by many years of experience. Recognition of a seizure's EEG pattern is extremely important in making the diagnosis of epilepsy in selected patients. Scalp-recorded interictal EEG study, neurologic history and examination, and brain imaging procedures (discussed next) may not always permit clear event classification. The potential disadvantages of video-EEG recordings include the cost of the study and hospitalization and the need for special resources and personnel. The EEG pat-

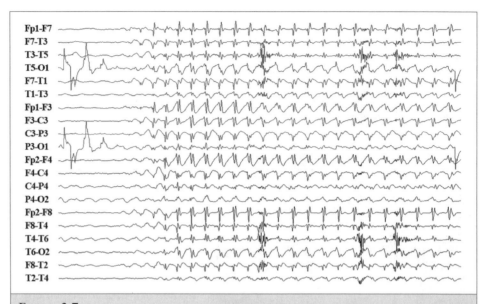

FIGURE 2.7
EEG pattern during an absence seizure in a child with staring spells.

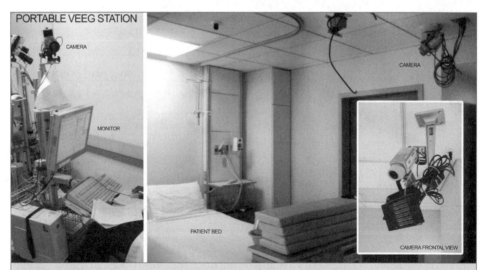

FIGURE 2.8
Video EEG set up in a patient's room with the camera installed on the ceiling (*right*) and a portable video EEG station (*left*).

terns may also be difficult to interpret because of artifacts related to movement and eye blinking. Finally, patients may not have a typical clinical event during video-EEG monitoring. However, in the majority of patients, the video-EEG study is very helpful, and it may be the definitive test for most patients.

Neuroimaging

Magnetic Resonance Imaging

Nearly all patients being evaluated for seizures or epilepsy require magnetic resonance imaging (MRI). An MRI machine uses a big magnet that, through a complicated set of changes, can make beautiful pictures of the body. The patient usually has to lie still inside a large tube or tunnel while the magnet scans his body (Figure 2.9). Most studies of the brain last about 30 to 40 minutes. The MRI machine can be quite noisy while it is scanning.

The MRI supplies detailed information about the structure or anatomy of the brain. It is highly sensitive for localizing strokes, tumors, birth defects, scar tissue from traumatic injury, and other abnormalities associated with seizures. In temporal lobe epilepsy, which is the most common type of epilepsy treated with surgery, shrinkage of a deep part of the temporal lobe (the *hippocampus*) can be seen. Sometimes, a contrast agent, *gadolinium*, is injected during the MRI as well. This contrast agent allows the neurolo-

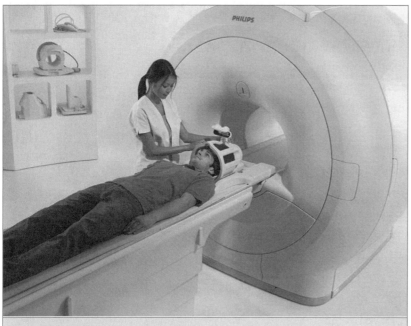

FIGURE 2.9
A MRI machine is shown with a patient being prepared for scanning.

gist to see certain details of the brain more clearly.

Because many studies have shown that MRI is the best technique we have to find the cause of seizures, it is the imaging procedure of choice in patients with epilepsy (Figure 2.10) MRI is very good at revealing common physical disturbances within the brain, such as head trauma, vascular malformations, and tumors (Figure 2.11). MRI is better and more specific than x-ray computed tomography (CT or CAT scan) in patients with seizure disorders. The MRI has an important role in identifying potential patients for *epilepsy surgery* and in planning the operation for the surgeon. The negative aspects of MRI include patient claustrophobia (afraid of small space), excess body size, and the presence of some foreign metallic objects (such as cardiac pacemakers and certain heart valves or aneurysm clips). The latter may not permit the MRI study. Dental work and minor surgical procedures (like suturing of scalp lacerations or paranasal sinus surgery) usually have little effect on the quality of an MRI.

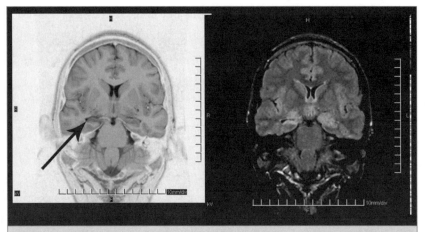

FIGURE 2.10
MRI shows medial temporal lobe atrophy in a patient with temporal lobe epilepsy.

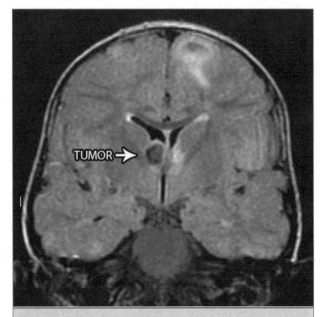

FIGURE 2.11
This MRI shows multiple lesions including a small tumor (*arrow*) in a patient with tuberous sclerosis.

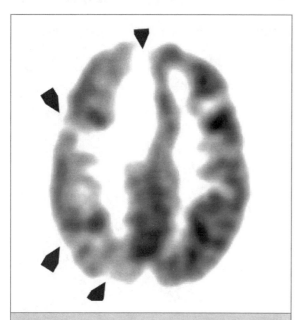

FIGURE 2.12
PET scan shows multiple regions (*arrows*) of low glucose uptake in a patient with epilepsy (courtesy of H Chugani, Detroit).

MRI is a painless technique, although it may be uncomfortable for people who suffer from claustrophobia. Claustrophobia can usually be managed through sedation or the use of an "open" MRI scanner that does not require the patient to be placed entirely within the MRI machine. Patients who are excessively large (both by body weight and shoulder width) may not fit into the tunnel of the typical MRI scanner. These patients may also be candidates for an open MRI scan. Unfortunately, open MRIs have lower resolution and may be less likely to find something wrong that the traditional tunnel-type scanner. Young children and adults with mental retardation may require general anesthesia to safely complete an MRI study. There are no known harmful side effects of MRI if the patients imaged do not have the contraindications noted earlier (metallic implants, etc.). MRI does not involve any radioactive substances. The benefits of MRI must be weighed against any potential risks in pregnant women.

Positron Emission Tomography

Positron emission tomography (PET) is a nuclear medicine imaging study that may be useful in identifying a localized abnormality in patients with partial epilepsy. This may assist the surgical planning in individuals being considered for *epilepsy surgery*. This test is not routine, and it should be used only if surgery is a consideration. Further information on PET is provided in Chapter 5 (Figure 2.12).

Single Photon Emission Computed Tomography

Single photon emission computed tomography (SPECT) is another nuclear medicine imaging study used in patients being considered for *epilepsy surgery* to identify a focal blood flow alteration that may indicate the location of the epileptic brain tissue. SPECT is more available than PET, but it is reserved mainly for patients who are considering surgery; it is discussed further in Chapter 5 (Figure 2.13).

CLINICAL APPLICATIONS OF DIAGNOSTIC STUDIES

Recurrent Spells

Patients may be referred for the evaluation and treatment of recurrent and unprovoked clinical spells. An estimated 20% of patients referred to comprehensive epilepsy programs for medically intractable "seizures" do not have epilepsy (Table 2.1). The issues to be considered in caring for these patients include diagnostic classification, potential causes, and treatment options. The neurologic history and examination, and routine EEG, indicate the classification of the seizure type and allow selection of an appropriate antiepileptic medication in about half the patients.

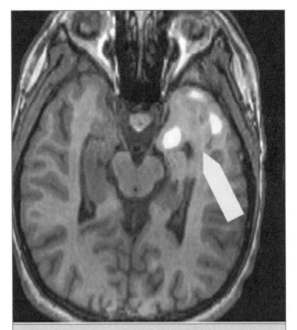

FIGURE 2.13
SISCOM subtraction ictal SPECT co-registered to MRI reveals a left temporal lobe blood flow change (arrow). The white areas represent increase blood flow changes.

Common events that are referred for diagnosis include potential psychological and physiologic nonepileptic disorders that involve sudden changes in behavior. Patients with an underlying psychiatric disease, such as depression, anxiety, or psychosis, may experience recurrent events that look like seizures. Psychogenic spells or *pseudoseizures* may be present in the absence of a major psychiatric disorder. It is not uncommon for patients with psychogenic events to have many normal EEG recordings, a remote history of emotional or sexual abuse, an unusual response to medication (increase in spells with the use of antiepileptic drugs), and unusual symptoms suggesting a behavioral disorder. The spells may be prolonged in duration and associated with headache, generalized pain, or crying. Importantly, the clinical features alone may be unclear in differentiating nonepileptic behavioral events from seizures. For that reason, video-EEG evaluation is needed for many of these patients.

Other nonepileptic events with episodic behavioral changes include cardiac disease, syncope, tremor, chemical dysfunction, and medication toxicity. These can be differentiated from psychogenic events through the use of laboratory testing and video-EEG.

Seizure Type Classification

A very important indication for video-EEG monitoring in patients with epilepsy is seizure classification (type). Classifying the seizure type in a patient with epilepsy is very important

---

TABLE 2.2

Summary of the International Classification of Epileptic Seizures

Commission on Classification, 1981

I.   Partial (focal, local) seizures
    A.   Simple partial seizures (consciousness not impaired)
        With motor symptoms
        With somatosensory or special sensory symptoms
        With autonomic symptoms
        With psychic symptoms
    B.   Complex partial seizures (with impairment of consciousness)
        B.1.   Beginning as simple partial seizures and progressing to impairment of consciousness
            With no other features
            With features as in I.A
            With automatisms
        B.2.   With impairment of consciousness at onset
            With no other features
            With features as in I.A
            With automatisms
    C.   Partial seizures secondarily generalized
II.   Generalized seizures (convulsive or nonconvulsive)
        Absence seizures
        Myoclonic seizures
        Clonic seizures
        Tonic seizures
        Tonic-clonic seizures
        Atonic seizures
III.   Unclassified epileptic seizures
IV.   Status epilepticus and provoked seizures

---

for choosing the correct drug treatment (Table 2.2). The routine EEG study and neurologic history may not always be able to determine the seizure type(s). One potential clinical problem is the patient with frequent convulsions (generalized tonic–clonic seizures) who may have either generalized or partial epilepsy. Classification of the exact epileptic condition will be used to determine what other tests are needed and the best medication to control the seizures. Some patients with periods of blank behavior may have absence, atypical absence (petit mal), or complex partial seizures (see Chapter 1). The introduction of so many new antiepileptic drugs has made diagnostic classification more important now than ever.

FREQUENTLY ASKED QUESTIONS

Q Do I have epilepsy when I experience a single seizure?

A The diagnosis of epilepsy is confirmed when a patient experiences two or more unprovoked seizures. Many individuals with a single seizure will not experience seizure recurrence. Approximately 10% of individuals will experience one or more seizures during their lifetime. The risk of recurrent seizures is greatest in patients with a history of a previous significant neurologic disorder (like a brain tumor), an abnormal MRI head study, an abnormal EEG that shows epileptiform activity, an abnormal neurologic examination that suggests a localized structural alteration in the brain, and a positive family history of epilepsy. One or more of these factors may increase the risk of seizure recurrence. Patients with a normal neurologic evaluation may be at lower risk of a second seizure. Patients who experience a single seizure should undergo an appropriate medical and neurologic evaluation. In the adult patient, this almost invariably means a brain MRI and EEG study will be performed. A cerebrospinal fluid examination may be indicated if the patient is thought to be at risk of meningitis (an infection in the spinal fluid and lining of the brain). The rationale for the use of antiepileptic medication is to lower the risk of seizure recurrence. There are conflicting findings regarding the use of antiepileptic drug therapy in patients who experience only a single seizure or very few seizures. The potential disadvantages include the potential for drug side effects, interaction with other medications, pregnancy-related complications, and the cost and expense associated both with the prescription and need for laboratory studies. Not uncommonly, the physician will individualize the need for antiepileptic drug therapy at the end of the diagnostic evaluation. The prevailing evidence suggests that many individuals who experience a single seizure do not require long-term antiepileptic medication.

Q **If my EEG is normal, do I have epilepsy?**

A Patients may have a single normal wake–sleep EEG and still have a seizure disorder. Approximately 50% to 90% of patients with epilepsy will have an abnormal EEG if multiple EEG recordings are performed. The yield of the routine EEG recording depends on multiple factors including the type of seizure activity, location of seizure onset, age of the patient, frequency of seizures, and presence of antiepileptic medication. The timing of the last seizure may affect the sensitivity of the EEG recording. The closer the EEG is done in relation to a seizure, the more likely the study will be abnormal. Use of additional scalp electrodes, a prolonged period for an EEG recording, and activation procedures (like hyperventilation and photic stimulation) may enhance the likelihood of recording a specific abnormality that indicates a seizure disorder. Selected individuals may have repetitively "normal" EEG recordings and still have a seizure disorder. The diagnosis of epilepsy requires the appropriate clinical history with supporting evaluation. In some instances, admission to an epilepsy monitoring unit for long-term EEG recordings may be necessary to confirm the diagnosis and initiate therapy.

Q **If the EEG and MRI are normal, should I receive antiepileptic medication for my seizure disorder?**

A Patients with epilepsy may have a normal routine EEG results and MRI scans. The decision regarding the use of medication in these patients depends on the clinical history and additional information. The diagnosis of epilepsy does not necessarily require an abnormal routine EEG and MRI. As discussed in Question 2, the EEG may be unremarkable, especially with only a single recording. MRI may demonstrate a structural abnormality associated with a partial seizure disorder. However, in a significant number of patients with partial or generalized epilepsy, the MRI does not reveal a specific alteration. The technique used for the MRI study is important. Your doctor should personally review the MRI to make certain the study has been done appropriately, and to see if, in the context of your particular history, a subtle abnormality is present. The decision regarding medical therapy in patients with normal EEG and MRI studies depends on the seizure type, the likely "mechanism" of seizure activity, and potential underlying cause(s). Subsequent EEG and MRI studies in selected patients may reveal abnormalities that may provide indispensable information concerning the cause of epilepsy, type of seizure disorder, and likely site of seizure onset.

Q What happens if I am admitted to the epilepsy monitoring unit for seizure classification and do not have a seizure?

A Patients are admitted to an epilepsy monitoring for two important reasons. The first is to classify seizure type. The second may be to localize the site of seizure onset prior to possible epilepsy surgery. To increase the likelihood of recording a seizure or spell, your antiepileptic medication may be discontinued or reduced. Other seizure-precipitating factors that may be used include sleep deprivation, photic stimulation, hyperventilation, and exercise using a treadmill or bicycle. The average duration for epilepsy monitoring is variable, and depends on a number of factors including the frequency of seizure activity. Prolonged EEG recordings made between the clinical spells (*interictal* EEG patterns) may be useful for diagnostic classification. The convergence of diagnostic studies (routine EEG, MRI) and the neurologic history-examination may also permit a presumptive diagnosis of epilepsy, despite the fact that you do not have a typical spell. Often this information may allow your doctor to determine the most likely effective antiepileptic drug therapy. Finally, in selected patients, further inpatient monitoring may need to be performed at another time to try to record seizure activity if the initial evaluation is nondiagnostic.

Q How can the doctor localize the site of seizure onset if the MRI is normal?

A Localization of epileptic tissue is particularly important in patients with medically refractory or intractable seizures being considered for surgical treatment. The EEG is the appropriate study to determine the site of seizure onset. MRI may demonstrate a structural lesion or abnormality that may indicate the cause of the seizure disorder and indirectly suggest the localization of the epileptic brain tissue. Video-EEG monitoring has been the "gold standard" to determine the classification of seizure type and the area of the brain involved in the seizure activity. The *ictal* EEG pattern (the pattern present during the habitual seizures) is pivotal to select candidates for the surgical treatment of intractable epilepsy. Most operative procedures (referred to commonly as *epilepsy surgery*) involve *resection* or removal of the epileptic brain tissue. In selected candidates, EEG recordings may be performed in the operating room (directly from the brain and not the scalp; this is referred to as *electrocorticography*). Not uncommonly, scalp-electrode EEG monitoring does not permit the exact localization of the site of seizure onset to determine the most effective operative procedure. *Chronic intracranial EEG monitoring* (placement of electrodes on the brain surface or in regions of the brain) is performed to record the habitual seizures and better localize the epileptic brain tissue. This requires a neurosurgical procedure to place the electrodes, and it is only performed after a comprehensive noninvasive evaluation. Other imaging studies are commonly performed in patients with a normal MRI when there is concern regarding the site of seizure onset in potential surgical candidates. PET, SPECT, or magnetic resonance spectroscopy (MRS) may be useful in guiding the presurgical evaluation.

My Notes

_____

_____

_____

_____

_____

_____

3

EPILEPSY TREATMENT

General Considerations

Key Points

▶ A single seizure may occur in any person under certain extreme provocations.

▶ It is important to prevent recurrent seizures because seizures can be associated with various injuries.

▶ Diagnosing the seizure type is important when choosing the best medication to prevent seizures.

▶ Once a medication is started, it should be started at a low dose and increased in small, slow steps.

▶ Studies show that approximately two-thirds of people who just started having seizures will stop having seizures with drug treatment.

▶ Certain forms of epilepsy are more likely to respond to treatment than others.

AS WE NOW UNDERSTAND, epilepsy is a condition characterized by recurrent unprovoked seizures, or at least one seizure in addition to a persistent tendency to develop additional seizures. This chapter focuses on the treatment of epilepsy to prevent recurrent seizures. Since most seizures stop by themselves, there is usually no need to treat individual seizures, unless they continue beyond 5 minutes. At present, no medication can eliminate the tendency for seizures altogether, unless the seizures are caused by an underlying treatable infectious or inflammatory condition. Discovering treatments to cure epilepsy, however is a strong focus of research. If a treatment is found that can permanently reverse the seizure tendency in patients (in the same way that an antibiotic can cure pneumonia), such a treatment could become very important.

This chapter discusses treatment decisions, beginning with the first seizure. It also discusses the duration of successful treatment, the management of recurrent seizures that do not respond to initial medications, and other various aspects of treatment.

SINGLE SEIZURES

Provoked Seizures

A single seizure may occur in any person when subjected to certain extreme provocations. For example, anyone may develop a seizure if exposed to certain toxic substances or if an extreme change in the mineral composition of their blood occurs. Single seizures may also occur in individuals who drink alcohol heavily on a regular basis and then suddenly stop drinking. In this setting, the tendency to have seizures is short-lasting. The seizures occur typically within 2 days of the last drink. A similar pattern may occur in individuals who suddenly stop taking certain sleeping pills or "nerve" medications. Although there could be a series of seizures, the tendency does not persist and, after the seizures have stopped, they do not keep coming back.

Provoked Seizures and Long-term Treatment

In the setting of a single seizure clearly provoked by a drug or a change in blood composition, correcting the underlying problem can eliminate the seizure tendency. Long-term treatment is only for the prevention of recurrent seizures. This is not usually necessary for provoked seizures, unless the underlying provoking factor cannot be easily corrected. In one study, the risk of an unprovoked seizure was only 13% after a short provoked seizure. However, if the first seizure was very long (known as *status epilepticus*), then the risk of an unprovoked seizure increased to about 41%.

Reasons for Treatment to Prevent Recurrent Seizures

It's important to prevent recurrent seizures because seizures can be associated with various injuries. Due to the risk of injury, recurrent seizures result in certain lifestyle restrictions, specifically restrictions on driving, on working in environments that could result in an injury in the event of a seizure, and on working at a job in which a seizure can be disruptive.

Recurrent seizures may also result in loss of brain cells if allowed to continue uncontrolled. Seizures may occasionally become more severe. For example, it is possible that after a mild complex partial seizure, the second seizure could be a more severe generalized tonic–clonic seizure.

Uncontrolled seizures may interfere with functioning. In particular, people with uncontrolled seizures frequently report difficulties with memory because seizures often involve parts of the brain (the temporal lobes) important for memory.

There is a small but definite risk of sudden unexpected death during seizures, but it has been demonstrated that this increased risk is largely eliminated if seizures are well controlled.

These factors do not all apply to every seizure type. It is well known that generalized absence seizures (frequently called *petit mal* seizures) do not cause cell loss in the brain. However, they do interfere with reaction time; people with generalized absence seizures will be restricted from driving and engaging in other potentially risky activities.

Risk of Recurrence and Treatment for a Single Unprovoked Seizure

When the first seizure is unprovoked or is related only to a mild provocation (such as sleep deprivation) that does not generally result in seizures in most individuals, then treatment may be considered. Studies indicate that a second seizure occurs in only 40% to 50% of people overall. If everybody with a single unprovoked seizure were to be treated, then a lot of people would be treated unnecessarily. As a result, doctors look into factors that can help predict who will have a second seizure.

Medical Tests before Treatment of a First Unprovoked Seizure

In most instances, when a decision has to be made about treatment, the neurologist needs a very good description of the seizures. This requires talking to a witness who has seen the seizure. Based on this description, the neurologist will decide if the seizure was indeed epileptic. Many conditions can imitate epileptic seizures (see Chapters 1 and 2). If it is decided that the seizure was indeed epileptic, the neurologist should explore past diseases or injuries that may have affected the brain and produced a tendency for seizures. Tests that the neurologist will obtain are described in Chapter 2.

Factors That Predict Recurrent Seizures

Individuals who are more likely to have recurrent seizures include people who have a structural abnormality in the brain (for example, an old injury such as scar, a tumor, or other *lesion*), people who have other members of their family with epilepsy, and people who have an abnormal EEG (Table 3.1). People with a single seizure who have none of these factors are much less likely to have another seizure, with odds of another seizure as low as one in four or one in three. However, the decision to start a new medication or not must involve the patient and the patient's

---

TABLE 3.1

Factors Predicting a Higher Risk of Another Seizure after a Single Seizure

▶ Cause of epilepsy—Abnormal brain structure or brain function as a cause of seizure (e.g., cerebral palsy, mental retardation)

▶ Abnormal electroencephalogram (EEG)

▶ Seizure type—Partial seizures predict greater likelihood of recurrence than generalized seizures (but this is not consistently found)

▶ Other factors found in some studies:
  – Seizure while asleep
  – Prior seizures with high fever
  – Weakness on one side of the body after the seizure

---

personal situation. Certain personal factors may make it wise to treat an individual with a low risk of another seizure, while other factors may make it worthwhile to withhold treatment in someone who has a high risk of another seizure. For example, a working adult may be at risk of losing his job if he has another seizure. Treatment may then be recommended for such an individual, even though the risk of recurrence is not high. On the other hand, treatment may be withheld in a child who is not working or driving, if the family is very concerned about the risk of side effects from medication or the effect that a medication may have on learning.

Risk of Seizure Recurrence after Two or More Seizures

If a second seizure occurs, then the risk that a third seizure will occur is almost three out of four. Once three seizures have occurred, approximately 81% of people will experience another seizure. The majority of recurrences will occur within the first year. Because of these statistics, treatment is almost always recommended after two or more seizures. However, some circumstances could make the decision to treat not so straightforward. For instance, if the seizures are several years apart, it may be hard to justify taking daily medications to prevent another seizure that may not happen for several years.

Medication Choices after a First Unprovoked Seizure

Many seizure medications are available for us to choose from. Although most of these medications have been proven effective, some have not been tested as stand-alone medications in people who just started having seizures (i.e., they have been tested only as additional medication and in patients whose seizures have been resistant to treatment). Therefore, not every epilepsy medication is appropriate for use as a first drug. Only some of the available medications have been com-

These case studies are real examples of the problems facing patients and doctors when decisions regarding treatment must be made.

Example 1. Single seizure during sleep.
A 13-year-old boy had a single seizure in sleep. His parents heard a noise and walked into his room to find him jerking from all extremities and producing a snorting noise. The next day, his pediatrician finds him completely normal. The neurologist also finds a completely normal neurologic examination. MRI of the brain and EEG are normal. The advantages and disadvantages of starting a seizure medication are discussed with the family. In this case, the risk of another seizure is probably around 30%. The child is not yet of driving age, and the risks of another seizure do not seem to be major. On the other hand, the family is concerned that medications may affect learning in school. All these factors tilt the balance toward not treating, but just observing the child for the possibility of another seizure.

Example 2. Single seizure in working adult.
A 35-year-old nurse has a seizure at work characterized by staring, lip smacking, and unresponsiveness for about 2 minutes. During that time, she picks repeatedly at the bed sheets of a patient. Testing shows that she has a normal MRI and a normal EEG. Neurologic examination is completely normal. There are no definite risk factors for epilepsy. The advantages and disadvantages of treatment are discussed with the patient. She feels that her job is at risk, and that another seizure may cause her to lose her job. Even though the risk of another seizure is low, the consequences seem to be too great, and the patient decides to start a medication.

Example 3. Adult with provoked single seizure.
A 40-year-old man awakens his wife at night with jerking of all extremities for about 1 minute, after which he is limp and unresponsive, with loud respirations. He goes back to sleep and has no memory of the event the next day. He had a severe head injury 5 years previously, resulting in weakness on the left side of the body ever since that injury. MRI shows a scar in the right brain with evidence of old injury. The EEG shows abnormal waves in the right frontal region of the brain. In this case, the risk that a second seizure will occur is greater than 50%. It seems quite advisable to start treatment.

pared with each other to see how effective they are and how well a patient can tolerate them. For example, the older medications such as carbamazepine (Tegretol/Carbatrol), phenytoin (Dilantin), primidone (Mysoline), and phenobarbital were compared in patients with partial seizures. It was very clear that primidone and phenobarbital were less well tolerated than the other medications, and therefore these are no longer recommended as first-line drugs. Among the new medications, those that have been properly tested for initial use include gabapentin (Neurontin), lamotrigine (Lamictal), topiramate (Topamax), and oxcarbazepine (Trileptal). Testing is in progress for other drugs. Because the U.S. Food and Drug Administration (FDA) has strict criteria for drug approval, it has only approved oxcarbazepine (Trileptal) and topiramate (Topamax) as first-line treatment.

Influence of Seizure Type on Choice of Medication

Diagnosing the seizure type is important when choosing the best medication to prevent seizures. Not all seizure types respond to the same medications. For example, generalized absence seizures respond to ethosuximide (Zarontin) and divalproex sodium (Depakote), but not to phenytoin (Dilantin), carbamazepine (Tegretol/Carbatrol), or phenobarbital, which are effective against partial seizures and generalized tonic–clonic seizures. As a result, it is very important to diagnose the seizure type and the form of epilepsy before choosing the most appropriate drug.

Considerations in Choosing the First Drug

Choosing the most appropriate drug takes into account many considerations. These considerations include age, gender, potential for becoming pregnant, other medical illnesses, other medications being used, and other factors. For example, several recent studies compared carbamazepine (Tegretol) and lamotrigine (Lamictal) in seniors with new-onset seizures and found that lamotrigine (Lamictal) was better tolerated in this age group. It is now established that exposure during pregnancy to divalproex (Depakote) is associated with an increased risk of birth defects; therefore, this drug may not be appropriate as a first choice in a woman intending to get pregnant soon. Many people with new-onset seizures have migraine headaches. Using one medication to treat both migraine and seizures is an attractive possibility that would certainly influence the choice of medication. Medication side effects also affect the choice. For example, in a person with a strong family history of kidney stones, topiramate (Topamax) may not be a good choice because it is associated with an increased risk of kidney stones. In a person who has a history of severe skin reaction, lamotrigine (Lamictal) may be avoided because it has a higher risk of serious skin rash.

Guidelines to Starting the First Medication

Once a medication is started, it should be started at a low dose and increased in small, slow steps. The principle "start low and go slow" is almost always wise, unless there is a rush to reach an effective level because the first seizure was particularly severe, or because several seizures have occurred within a short time. After a single seizure, it is hard to know how much medication is needed to prevent subsequent seizures. It may therefore be wise to increase the dose to an amount known to be effective from experience with other individuals. In people who have had repeated seizures, this may not be the case: As the dose is slowly increased, the seizures may stop, even if the dose is much smaller than what is well known to be generally effective.

If there is a need to reach a protective dose very rapidly, some medications are not a good choice. For example, lamotrigine (Lamictal) cannot be started and increased rapidly because we know this increases the risk of allergic rash. Topiramate (Topamax) cannot be increased rapidly because it can result in difficulty concentrating.

MONITORING AND OPTIMIZING TREATMENT

Monitoring Treatment with Blood Tests

Two forms of blood tests are used to monitor people taking seizure medications. One measures the level of the medication in the blood—the *drug levels*. The other test measures blood count, liver enzymes, and mineral blood composition because these may be affected by treatment. It is generally felt that measuring the level of medication in the blood is not essential, although it is helpful as a reference point once the target dose is reached. This may help show a doctor how much leeway there is with increasing the dose, and it may also serve as a reference point should seizures recur or problems appear later on—the drug level can be obtained at the point in question and compared with the initial level. This comparison could help explain what caused the seizures to recur or what caused side effects to appear. For older medications, doctors sometimes have a good idea about what level is most likely to be effective and what level is most likely to cause side effects.

However, it is a mistake to make adjustments based on the blood level of a medication alone. Enough variability exists between people that a blood level effective for one may be ineffective for another, or a blood level that is toxic for one can be well tolerated by another. For most medications, the blood-level test does not need to be repeated at set periods. For most seizure medications, the change in blood level is proportional to the change in dose. For example, if the dose is increased by 25%, one expects the level of drug in the blood to increase by about 25%. However, there is one important exception to this rule, and that exception is phenytoin (Dilantin), one of the most frequently used medications for seizures. Neurologists must be very careful about how fast they increase the dose of phenytoin (Dilantin) because it builds up rapidly in the bloodstream. A doctor may use very small dose increases of phenytoin (Dilantin) when it is close to the range that is most often effective.

For the older medications, such as phenytoin (Dilantin), carbamazepine (Tegretol or Carbatrol), divalproex sodium (Depakote), and phenobarbital, we have a fairly good idea of the effective blood-level range. For the newer medications, the effective range is generally not well established. When a new medication level is obtained, the laboratory provides a comparison with the usual range seen on doses that were used in research studies (rather than the known most effective range). One of the newer antiepileptic drugs, lamotrigine (Lamictal), has such a general range defined; above this range, it is likely that side effects will appear. Birth control pills and pregnancy markedly reduce the level of lamotrigine (Lamictal) in the blood. Therefore, checking blood levels of lamotrigine (Lamictal) after becoming pregnant or after starting birth control pills may be important for appropriate adjustments in the dose.

Checking and Monitoring Blood Count and Liver Enzymes

Some seizure medications (particularly the older ones) have been associated with occasional changes in liver enzymes or blood count. Other medications may reduce sodium level. When starting these medications, it may be reasonable to check these levels at baseline and then once or twice after treatment is initiated, from 3 to 6 months after starting treatment. For individuals in whom these values do not change, it is not necessary to continue these blood tests.

Optimizing Treatment and Determining That a Drug Has Failed

If the diagnosis of epileptic seizures is very clearly established and an appropriate medication has been started, but seizures continue to occur, certain steps should be considered before concluding that the medication has failed. The possibility should be considered that the medication dose has not been pushed to an optimal level. So much variation exists among individuals that a dose effective for one person may be ineffective for another. This could be because the medication was less well absorbed or because of rapid breakdown of the medication in the patient's system. Thus, if no side effects are present, it is usually appropriate to continue increasing the dose as long as seizures are not yet controlled. A blood level can help clarify the situation. However, this is true only for some medications. For individuals who are clearly resistant to the maximum tolerated dose of a medication, a change in treatment must be considered. Once at least two drugs have been failed in this manner, and if the diagnosis and the classification of epilepsy are identified beyond doubt, then the possibility of surgical treatment should be considered for patients who have partial epilepsy. If a well-defined lesion or *hippocampal sclerosis* (a condition

---

Example 4. Optimizing treatment with a new drug.
A young man is taking 600 mg per day of lamotrigine (Lamictal) and still having one seizure every 2 months. He is not experiencing any side effects. His physician is worried that these seizures continue despite a dose of Lamictal that is higher than he normally prescribes. He obtains a blood level, which is 4 micrograms per milliliter (mcg/mL). Studies suggest that some people can continue to derive benefit from Lamictal up to a level of 20 mcg/mL. A level of 4 mcg/mL is an indication that there is a lot of leeway for increasing the dose. The appropriate step is to increase the dose of lamotrigine. This may not need a blood level, and the dose could be increased as long as no adverse experiences occur. However, the blood level helps increase confidence in the appropriateness of increasing the medication dose.

with cell loss and scarring affecting the hippocampus, a structure in the temporal lobe that is a common source of seizures) is present, then surgical treatment can be highly effective and should be considered early.

DETERMINING EFFECTIVENESS OF TREATMENT

Studies show that approximately two-thirds of people who just started having seizures will stop having seizures with drug treatment. Thus, approximately one-third may continue to have seizures and would thus be considered as having *refractory epilepsy*.

Defining Good Seizure Control

Only the complete absence of seizures can be considered a good end-point of treatment. Even though some individuals may be pleased to have only one seizure every 2 months when they used to have seizures every day, this is not satisfactory seizure control. *Any* persistent seizures are associated with the risks and restrictions listed earlier.

Reversible Causes of Treatment Failure

When seizures continue, it is essential to search for factors that may explain why treatment is failing. Some of these factors can be easily reversed. For example, sleep deprivation may be a cause of seizures not responding to treatment. This is particularly true in a form of epilepsy called *juvenile myoclonic epilepsy*. Evidence suggests that *sleep apnea*, which is a very common condition, particularly in overweight men, may cause sleep to be of poor quality and therefore may imitate the effect of sleep deprivation. This can cause seizures to be resistant to treatment. Treatment may also fail because of the use of recreational drugs or certain medications that can trigger seizures. In some individuals, an excessive intake of caffeine can result in breakthrough seizures. The effective treatment of epilepsy requires taking seizure medications regularly. Missing doses can reduce the medication blood level to the point at which the medication is not sufficient to protect from seizures. It is also possible that the drug has not been given a fair chance. Before a medication trial is considered to have failed, it is essential that the dose be pushed to the maximum amount tolerated. The dose necessary to stop seizures may be higher for some than for others. In the case of a medication like phenytoin (Dilantin), it is easy to totally skip the effective dose by making dose increases that are too large. Therefore, it is important to use small steps while exploring the dose that will control seizures eventually. It is also possible that the medication chosen is not appropriate. This is why it is essential to have a clear idea of the type of seizures present before starting treatment. Finally, it is also possible that the seizures are not epileptic, or that the patient has both epileptic and nonepileptic seizures; nonepileptic seizures will usually not respond to seizure medications. Even after accounting for these factors, approximately one-third of patients will continue to have seizures despite the best medical treatment.

Predicting Response to Treatment

Certain forms of epilepsy are more likely to respond to treatment, and others are more likely to be resistant to treatment. For example, patients with genetic epilepsies (who had no other neurologic problem in addition to epilepsy) are more likely to be seizure-free with treatment. Patients with hippocampal scarring are less likely to be seizure-free and, if they are seizure-free, they are more likely to need more than one seizure medication. Because epilepsy with hippocampal sclerosis is very effectively treated with surgery, this should be considered early in these patients (see Chapter 5).

Likelihood of Complete Seizure Control with First and Subsequent Medications

One important study showed that approximately one-half of patients stopped having seizures with the first drug tried, but only 13% with the second drug. If the first drug failed because of side effects rather than lack of efficacy, then the chance of the second drug being effective is no different from the chance of the first drug. However, if the first drug failed because of lack of efficacy, then the chance of the next drug being effective is less. In the same study, after failing the first and second drug, only 1% of patients became seizure free with a third drug, and 3% became seizure free by combining two drugs. Therefore, failing two drugs seems to indicate a high chance of refractory epilepsy.

MANAGING RECURRENT SEIZURES AND REFRACTORY EPILEPSY

Once two drugs have been failed, it becomes likely that the epilepsy is going to be difficult to control. This is true if the drugs have failed despite using an adequate dose and without causing unacceptable side effects. When the drugs fail because of bad side effects only, the chances are better that another drug without side effects will work. At this point, it is important to reevaluate the condition. Before deciding that treatment has failed, it is important to consider all the possible explanations listed earlier. If the drug has been appropriately pushed to the maximum dose tolerated, and if lifestyle factors (such as sleep deprivation, poor-quality sleep, recreational drugs, other medications, and excess caffeine) are excluded, the possibility should be considered that the drugs failed because the seizures are nonepileptic. If that is a possibility, then it becomes important to perform long-term video and EEG (V-EEG) monitoring. This test is designed to record seizures and analyze them for definitive diagnosis.

Adding a Second Drug versus Switching to Another Drug

Most neurologists will try another drug before combining two drugs. (The use of one medication at a time is referred to as *monotherapy*. The use of two or more drugs in combination is referred to as *polytherapy*.) However, no evidence suggests that monotherapy is more effective than polytherapy. If the first drug failed because of complete lack of efficacy, then it is most appropriate to switch to another. However, if the first drug was effective but not completely, then adding a second drug may be quite appropriate. Some drugs have not been sufficiently tested as stand-alone treatments and are best used in combination with another drug. It should be noted that if the decision is made to switch to another monotherapy (single drug), the switch usually involves adding the second drug before removing the first. If, in the process, the patient becomes seizure-free while still on both drugs, the neurologist may hesitate to remove the first drug, and *dual* or *polytherapy* may then result.

Many factors must be considered in the choice of the next drug. If the previous drug failed because of side effects, the doctor may want to consider a drug that does not share the same side effects as the first. If the previous drug failed because of lack of efficacy, then some doctors may consider another drug with a different mechanism of action. This approach, however, has a theoretical basis not proven in practice.

Advantages of Monotherapy versus Polytherapy

It is the rule that many medications for epilepsy are best tolerated when used alone. Using drugs in combination increases the chance of extra side effects and increases the chance of interaction between drugs. Early on in the treatment of refractory epilepsy, most neurologists will try to stick with one drug. However, if the drug currently used has produced an excellent but incomplete benefit, the possibility could be considered of adding another agent rather than completely replacing the existing drug. One study that compared these two approaches did not clearly identify one approach as superior to the other. However, when using two drugs in combination, the selection of the add-on drug must be made carefully. In addition, it may be wise to avoid adding a drug that has a similar mechanism of action because this may increase the chances of extra side effects. For example, it is well known that using lamotrigine (Lamictal) and carbamazepine (Tegretol) together can increase the risk of blurred vision, double vision, or dizziness.

Occasionally, however, the interaction of two medications could be favorable, such that they complement each other's action. For example, one study suggested that combining lamotrigine (Lamictal) and divalproex (Depakote) might produce an incremental benefit that is greater than the benefit of the two drugs taken separately. This is an appealing concept, but one that has not been clearly proven effective in practice.

It is usually desirable not to exceed two medications at the same time. However, there are instances where the epilepsy is so resistant that the doctor is forced to add a third medication. In these instances, he may consider removing one of the previous two medications, but this is not always possible. The interactions of these medications should be always taken into consideration.

After two or three failed medication trials, it is important to consider if epilepsy surgery is a good option (Figure 3.1). For that purpose, special testing will be needed (see Chapter 5).

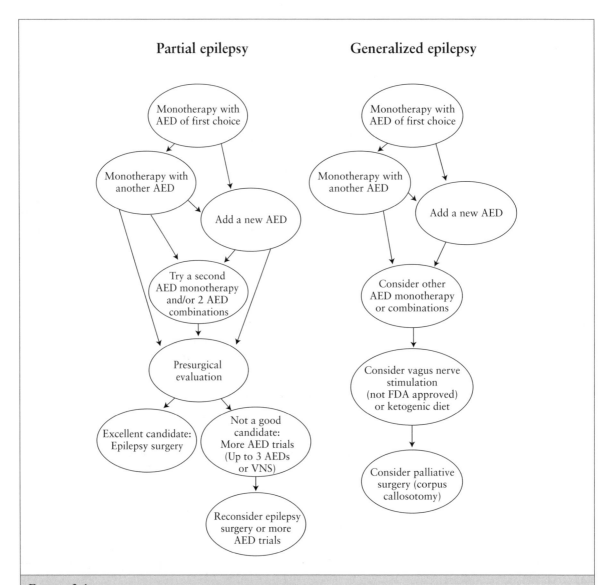

FIGURE 3.1

General guidelines for treatment steps. Vertical position generally reflects the order in which options are considered (higher position considered first). In this algorithm, it is assumed that the diagnosis is secure. The diagnosis must be confirmed with V-EEG early on, after the failure of no more than two drugs.

AED, antiepileptic drug; VNS, vagus nerve stimulation; FDA, Food and Drug Administration

Example 5. Managing refractory epilepsy.

A 24-year-old man started having seizures at age 19. These begin with a butterfly sensation in the pit of the stomach that rises to the throat, at which point he loses awareness and is noted to have lip smacking and picking movements with his right hand. After the seizure, he is tired for several minutes. He was started on one seizure medication that controlled his seizures completely for 2 years. Then, seizures started again and did not respond to increasing the dose of his medication. The dose was increased to the point at which he developed dizziness and excessive sleepiness. He wants to know what should he do next. His EEG shows abnormal waves in the right temporal lobe. His MRI shows right hippocampal scarring.

This patient most probably needs a change in treatment. He can be switched to a different drug, or another drug could be added to his current regime. Early on, at this stage of treatment, most neurologists would probably switch to another drug.

If the second drug does not work, even though it was pushed to high levels, then this patient should consider surgical treatment. The pattern of the seizures and the results of the EEG and the MRI suggest that he may be an excellent candidate for surgery. Epilepsy surgery will give him a 70% to 80% chance of being seizure-free.

AVOIDING AND DEALING WITH MEDICATION SIDE EFFECTS

Every medication has a potential for side effects that may affect a variable proportion of patients taking that medication. It is important for the patient and his physician to discuss the most common side effects of every medication before starting it. Some individuals are particularly susceptible to developing certain side effects. For example, people who have a tremor before starting treatment should know that using a medication such as divalproex (Depakote) or lamotrigine (Lamictal) might increase the tremor. Similarly, people who have problems with word finding may need to avoid topiramate (Topamax), which can cause speech difficulties.

Certain types of side effects can be managed without changing medications. For example, an inability to sleep that develops with lamotrigine (Lamictal) may be managed by changing the timing of the doses. Instead of taking the last dose at bedtime, it may be taken with supper or even as early as lunch. Some side effects occur 1 or 2 hours after taking a dose and last for only 30 minutes to 2 hours, linked to the timing of the medication dose. This is probably related to the medication level peaking in the blood. Such a side effect may be managed by splitting the dose in two or by taking the medication with food, which usually evens out the blood level peak. Because of this phenomenon, it may be advantageous to give the largest dose at bedtime (provided the medication does not interfere with sleep). Several medications are or soon will be available in extended-release preparation. Such a preparation may help smooth out the blood level fluctuations and provide both reduced side effects and greater efficacy throughout the day. Some side effects tend to disappear with the passage of time. This is particularly true of side effects that are mild to start with. One example is mild drowsiness.

Other side effects may be treated with supplements or medications. This is usually not a good idea unless the medication has produced excellent seizure control. For example, hair loss seen with divalproex (Depakote) may be helped by supplementing the diet with zinc and selenium. The excessive tiredness sometimes encountered with divalproex (Depakote) has been helped in some cases by the addition of L-carnitine. There is also anecdotal evidence that the mood swings sometimes encountered with levetiracetam (Keppra) can at times be helped by the addition of vitamin B_6.

In many instances, reducing the dose of the medication may take care of the side effects without losing seizure control. If seizures recur with dose reduction, the dose can be reduced for a while, then another attempt can be made at increasing it. Some side effects require stopping the medication, particularly if the side effects are severe and are not helped by reducing the dose. This is particularly true if the medication also did not control the seizures.

Predicting and Preventing Serious Complications from Medications

Several seizure medications also have the potential for rare, serious complications. These rare complications are difficult to predict. Sometimes, it is possible to identify people who are at risk for these adverse reactions. For example, the drug felbamate (Felbatol) is associated with a risk of bone marrow failure (aplastic anemia), which is often lethal. It is known that people who have baseline immune conditions, such as lupus, are at increased risk of developing this complication, and these individuals should not be started on this drug.

STOPPING MEDICATIONS

The treatment of epilepsy is not necessarily lifelong. Some forms of epilepsy are known to recover spontaneously, and it is therefore quite appropriate to consider removing treatment after seizures have been controlled for a period of time. In children, the longest waiting period before considering stopping seizure medications is 2 years. In adults, most neurologists wait longer before stopping seizure medications.

Reasons to Consider Stopping Medications

In some individuals, some medications may reduce concentration and learning, cause sleepiness or tiredness, or cause other bothersome side effects. Some patients also report changes in sexual function. In addition, some medications may have long-term effects, such as weight gain or reduced bone density. Because of these possible effects, a neurologist may favor removing medications if they are no longer necessary. However, it may be difficult to tell if or when the medication is no longer necessary.

Risk of Seizure Return after Stopping Medication

The risk always remains that seizures may come back after stopping seizure medications. Estimates of the risk of seizure recurrence after stopping seizure medications have varied. It is estimated that about 30% of patients will have seizure recurrence within 2 years of stopping medications. However, this depends on many factors.

A recurrence of seizures is more likely in people whose seizures are due to brain injury (Table 3.2). It is also more likely that seizures will come back if they started in adolescence, as opposed to childhood. In addition, an abnormal EEG at the time of stopping medications makes it more likely that seizures will come back. We can now predict that certain forms of epilepsy are unlikely to disappear.

The decision to stop medications depends on more than just the calculated risk of seizure recurrence. The doctor and patient should discuss the potential impact of a seizure on work and life in general. For example, a mother who has to drive her children to school every day should probably not plan on coming off seizure medications any time soon. The same would be true of a man whose job necessarily involves operating a forklift. If a patient decides to go ahead with medication withdrawal, it is best to plan for a time when driving can be avoided. Most neurologists will suggest not driving for 3 to 6 months in association with medication withdrawal. Medication withdrawal is much easier to consider in children who are not driving yet.

TABLE 3.2

Factors That Predict a Higher Risk of Another Seizure after Stopping Seizure Medications

▶ Cause of epilepsy—Abnormal brain structure or brain function as a cause of epilepsy (e.g., mental retardation or cerebral palsy)

▶ Abnormal electroencephalogram (EEG)

▶ Epilepsy starting in adolescence or adulthood has a greater risk than epilepsy starting in childhood

▶ Juvenile myoclonic epilepsy has a high risk of seizures after stopping medications

▶ Other factors found in some studies:
  – History of status epilepticus (continuous seizure activity)
  – Seizures that were frequent before they were controlled
  – History of epilepsy in other members of the family

> **Example 6. Deciding to stop seizure medications.**
>
> A 16-year-old boy had seizures starting at the age of 12 in which he lost consciousness first then had jerking of all extremities. These seizures came quickly under control with one seizure medication, and he has been seizure-free for 2 years. He is eager to start driving as soon as possible, and hates to take his medication. In fact, he often misses his morning dose, and has not had any problems with that. His MRI is normal. His first EEG showed epileptic discharges in one frontal lobe, but his EEG at age 16 was normal. This may be the ideal situation to consider medication withdrawal. This should probably be done before the patient starts driving. There is a suggestion that the epileptic condition may have resolved, since the EEG has become normal and no seizure occur when he misses his medication. It is probably best not to start driving until at least 3 months after coming off the medication.

Duration of Medication Withdrawal

It is the usual practice to stop a medication very gradually, usually over 3 to 6 months. However, one study showed no difference in outcome between *tapering* the medication over 6 weeks and over 9 months. If the patient is taking two medications, one medication should be slowly removed first, before the second medication is tapered.

The majority of individuals whose seizures return with removal of seizure medications will become seizure-free again after medications are restarted. However, some patients will continue to have seizures that can no longer be controlled. It is not totally clear if this was going to happen anyway, or if this is the result of stopping the medications.

FREQUENTLY ASKED QUESTIONS

Q I have had one seizure. Should I be treated?

A At present, the purpose of medication treatment is to prevent more seizures from happening. If the seizure was clearly provoked by a cause that is no longer present, then treatment is not necessary. For example, if the seizure is due to a very low sodium level, which is now corrected, treatment is not necessary. If the seizure occurred without provocation, then treatment could be advisable, and the pros and cons of treatment should be discussed with your neurologist. Overall, a second seizure occurs in only 40% to 50% of patients. People who have a normal neurologic examination, normal MRI scan of the brain, and normal EEG have a lower risk of seizure recurrence. They may consider not receiving any treatment. However, the decision may also depend on personal factors. For example, if there is a serious risk of job loss in the event of another seizure, this may affect the decision to treat.

Q Why is it important to prevent repeated seizures?

A It is important to prevent seizures if a high risk exists that another seizure may occur. The reasons include the following:

- ▶ Recurrent seizures could become more severe.
- ▶ Direct or indirect physical injury may result from a seizure.
- ▶ Loss of brain cells may occur from repeated severe seizures.
- ▶ Sudden death may occur rarely with severe seizures.
- ▶ Seizures can be associated with injury.
- ▶ Seizures result in legal restrictions on driving.

Q Now that I have been seizure-free for 6 months, I would like to come off seizure medications. Can I?

A It is recommended that treatment for seizures should continue for at least 2 years. Evidence suggests that the risk of seizure recurrence may be higher if medication is stopped earlier than that. Even after 2 years of no seizures on treatment, the risk is always present that seizures will come back after treatment is stopped, with approximately one-third of people having seizure recurrence. The risk of seizure recurrence can be predicted to some extent by the type and cause of epilepsy, the neurologic examination, and the result of EEG testing. For example, the risk of seizure recurrence in people with juvenile myoclonic epilepsy is very high, such that it is best not to stop treatment at any time.

Q Should I have blood tests every 3 months because I take a seizure medication?

A Routine blood testing is usually not necessary, except for some specific medications. Drug levels are usually not useful as a routine test. Drug levels can be useful if they answer a specific question. A drug level is useful:

- ▶ For future reference in a patient who is seizure-free
- ▶ To help explain lack of response at a high medication dose, and explore how much leeway there is for increasing the dose
- ▶ To help explain side effects at a low dose
- ▶ To monitor a known interaction for dose adjustment (for example, lamotrigine (Lamictal) dose changes may be needed after a birth control pill is added)

Q I am still having seizures! Why is the drug not working?

A Not all patients with epilepsy become seizure-free with treatment. Approximately one-third continue to have seizures despite the best treatment. After failing one medication, there is a fair chance that a second medication will work. However, when two medications have not worked, the chance of complete seizure cessation with a third medication becomes much smaller. When seizures are resistant to treatment, it is most important to verify that the attacks being treated are indeed epileptic seizures. It is also important to verify that the seizure type and form of epilepsy have been correctly diagnosed and treated with the most appropriate drug. Inpatient V-EEG monitoring is generally essential for answering these questions. If the seizures are indeed epileptic and are correctly diagnosed and treated, factors such as sleep deprivation, substance abuse, or the use of another medication that can trigger seizures must be explored and corrected.

My Notes

_____

_____

_____

_____

_____

_____

_____

_____

4

ANTIEPILEPTIC DRUGS

Medications and Side Effects

Key Points

▶ The goal of medication is to achieve the best seizure control possible, with few to no side effects.

▶ So far, no medication can cure epilepsy; AEDs work instead by suppressing seizure activity.

▶ Many antiepileptic medications have an established *therapeutic level*—the level at which a medication has been shown to control seizures and not produce adverse side effects.

▶ All medications have the potential of causing adverse side effects, and each drug will come with a long list of potential problems.

THERE ARE MANY WAYS TO TREAT EPILEPSY, but antiepileptic drugs (AEDs) remain the mainstay of treatment. When a firm diagnosis of epilepsy is made, treatment using antiepileptic medication is usually started either immediately or within days. Your doctor will prescribe a medication based on multiple factors, such as epilepsy and seizure type, age, gender, significant medical history, the side effect profile of each medication, as well as the cost of the drug. The goal of medication is to achieve the best seizure control possible, with few to no side effects (unwanted, bad effects).

The majority of people with epilepsy, over 50%, will achieve this goal. But, for others, seizure control will be more difficult and may require multiple medication trials, or the use of more than one medication at the same time. Some 20% to 30% of people with epilepsy will experience partial control of seizures, while approximately 20% will remain *refractory* (resistant) to medication.

More than a dozen antiepileptic medications currently are available, with more being developed and tested every day. This gives an individual and her doctor more options and a better chance at controlling epilepsy today, as compared to 10 or 15 years ago.

When a new drug is started, your doctor will provide a schedule to follow, as well as information about the possible side effects or problems that could occur with the medicine. Most drugs must be started gradually, increasing the dose a little at a time. Other drugs can be started more quickly. Slowly increasing a dose, which is called *titration*, usually gives your system a chance to get used to the medicine. This leads to fewer side effects and, in some instances, less chance of safety problems such as allergic reactions. Therefore, it's very important to make sure that your doctor's instructions are clear, and that you can follow them exactly. If, even when following instructions, some problem or side effect occurs, notify your doctor. Sometimes, these problems can be solved with a modification to the titration schedule, but in other cases a different drug will be substituted. Usually, after titration, the medication dose will be increased until seizure control is achieved. This will mean additional increases each time a seizure occurs. Often, the higher the dose, the better the seizures can be controlled. Therefore, your doctor may continue to increase your medication until or unless side effects occur. Side effects are the sign that another drug choice will be necessary. During this period, it is very important for doctor and patient to have open communication, because changes in drug dose or selection will depend entirely on the seizures and medication effects.

CONTINUED TREATMENT

Doctors typically use one medication, at the lowest dose possible, to treat seizures. Using one drug alone is called *monotherapy*. If a medication fails, either because it failed to control seizures or because it caused side effects, a second medication may be added. Some doctors will wean the first medication while starting the new one, while others will prefer to continue both medicines, at least for a while, to see what happens with seizure control. The use of one medication is often preferable for multiple reasons: it's cheaper, easier for increased *compliance* (taking the correct medicine at the scheduled time), and produces fewer side effects and interactions between medicines. While most people with epilepsy can be controlled using a single medication, patients with difficult-to-control seizures may require two or more medications (known as *polytherapy* or *polypharmacy*).

HOW ANTIEPILEPTIC DRUGS WORK

Some AEDs are listed in Table 4.1. The *mechanism of action*, or how these medicines work to stop seizures, is often not known completely. Some medications work by preventing epileptic cells from firing abnormally while leaving the normal firing of brain cells unchanged. Because seizures are thought to be a sign of brain-cell overexcitation, some medications increase *inhibitory pathways*, by increasing a normally occurring brain chemical called *gamma-amino butyric acid* (GABA). Other medications decrease *excitatory pathways* through systems that use the excitatory chemical *glutamate*. Other AEDs work in more than one way.

So far, no medication can cure epilepsy; AEDs work instead by suppressing seizure activity. That means they have to be constantly present in the brain. After a medication is taken by mouth, it is passed through the stomach and absorbed by the small intestine, then transported to the bloodstream, and eventually it reaches the brain. Some medicines leave the body when they are broken down (*metabolized*) by the liver. Others are not metabolized by the liver, but are cleared from the body by the kidneys, through the urine. When a medication is metabolized, a chemical product can result. This chemical, if active, can also help control seizures, or it can contribute to

---

TABLE 4.1

Common Antiepileptic Drugs

Carbamazepine (Tegretol, Tegretol XR, Carbatrol)	Phenobarbital (Luminal)
Ethosuximide (Zarontin)	Phenytoin (Dilantin, Phenytek)
Felbamate (Felbatol)	Primidone (Mysoline)
Gabapentin (Neurontin)	Pregabalin (Lyrica)
Lacosamide (Vimpat)	Rufinamide (Banzel)
Lamotrigine (Lamictal)	Tiagabine (Gabitril)
Levetiracetam (Keppra, Keppra XR)	Topiramate (Topamax)
Oxcarbazepine (Trileptal)	Valproate (Depakote, Depakene)
	Zonisamide (Zonegran)

side effects. People metabolize medicines at different rates. So, some people will need higher doses than others.

BLOOD LEVELS

After a medication is ingested, it reaches a maximum level in the bloodstream within a certain amount of time, usually between 30 minutes and 6 hours. After that, the amount of medication in the bloodstream gradually drops. Since the bloodstream delivers medication to the brain, the amount getting to the brain will in most cases drop at about the same rate. If the level of medication in the brain drops too far, it may no longer be able to protect against a seizure. The amount of time it takes for the medication level to drop to half the amount of the peak level, is called its *half-life*. The half-life of a medication can be short, intermediate, or long. A medication with a short half-life must be taken more frequently to maintain a constant level in the bloodstream and brain, while a medication with a long half-life can be dosed at less frequent intervals. For most drugs, a blood test can measure the amount of medication in the bloodstream. This is called a *drug level*.

Many antiepileptic medications have an established *therapeutic level*—the level at which a medication has been to shown to control seizures and not produce adverse side effects. The therapeutic levels should be used as a guide only. Many people have good seizure control at what is considered low or *subtherapeutic* levels, or at high or *toxic* levels. Similarly, some patients experience side effects despite levels within the therapeutic range. Drug levels are routinely checked when a new medication is initiated, when a dose is adjusted, when there is a change in seizure frequency, or when adverse side effects are experienced. The levels should be checked at the same time of day, usually prior to the first dose of the day, when the level is at its lowest also known as the *trough level*. Knowing what the level is may help the doctor understand how fast the drug is being metabolized. Once a patient has stabilized on a drug regimen, the doctor will have a good idea of the right level of the medicine needed to control their seizures. If a *breakthrough seizure* or side effects occurs, it is important to get a level to see if it is higher or lower than expected.

MEDICATION SIDE EFFECTS

All medications have the potential of causing adverse side effects, and each drug will come with a long list of potential problems. These side effects, seen listed in a physician's desk reference or on a pamphlet received from your doctor or pharmacy, are the problems that *may* occur from taking a specific medication. Medications have different effects on different people. Side effects may be dose related (caused by high drug levels). If multiple medications are used, adverse side effects may be caused by the combination of medications rather than either drug alone. If they occur, most side effects are easily managed by adjusting the dosage of the medication or changing the time a medication is taken. If side effects are persistent and severe, withdrawal of the medication may be necessary. Antiepileptic medication should never be stopped abruptly, because this could lead to increased seizure severity and frequency, and possibly *status epilepticus* (continuous seizure activity), which is a medical emergency. If side effects are intolerable, it is best to consult your doctor, who will be able to give advice on how to adjust medication safely.

Idiosyncratic adverse effects are characterized by unusual responses to a drug and are not related to dose or drug level. These adverse effects can include an allergic reaction, inflammation of the liver or pancreas, or a problem with the blood cells. Symptoms associated with idiosyncratic adverse effects can include rash, fever, enlarged lymph nodes, unusual bleeding or bruising, severe stomach pain, nausea and vomiting, or a change in skin color. While many side effects are more of a nuisance and easily dealt with by dose adjustments, idiosyncratic reactions are considered serious, and the prescribing doctor must be notified immediately.

BRAND-NAME VERSUS GENERIC DRUGS

Every drug has a chemical (*generic*) name as well as one or several *brand* names (given in parentheses in this book), which are specific to the company that markets the drug. A drug may also have different *formulations*, such as liquid, solid, sprinkle, immediate-release, or long-acting. Unless you discuss it with your doctor, you should take the same brand and formulation consistently, since switching might change the amount of drug that is released, or the timing of release, and lead to swings in blood levels.

We've listed the common drugs for epilepsy here, and described them in detail, including the seizure types that the drug is commonly prescribed for, as well as common dose-related and idiosyncratic side effects, and common drug interactions to look out for. This list is not meant to be exhaustive. Each drug should be discussed with your doctor before starting it.

Carbamazepine (Tegretol, Tegretol XR, Carbatrol)

▶ Used for simple partial seizures, complex partial seizures, and generalized tonic–clonic seizures. Carbamazepine may cause absence, atypical absence, and myoclonic seizures to worsen.
▶ Common side effects:
 ▷ Double vision, headache, nausea, incoordination, drowsiness, difficulty concentrating, and dizziness are the most frequently reported side effects at the start of treatment. These side effects usually improve as the body adjusts to the medication or the dose is lowered.
▶ Rare less serious side effects, which may or may not require discontinuation:
 ▷ *Hyponatremia* (low sodium level), *leucopenia* (decrease of white blood cells).

▶ Rare serious side effects that usually require discontinuation:
  ▷ Liver failure, bone marrow failure, drug-related rash, and hypersensitivity.
▶ Potential long-term effects:
  ▷ Carbamazepine has an effect on the liver (*enzyme induction*) that speeds the metabolism of other substances. This may increase the metabolism of vitamin D, which can contribute to *osteopenia* (a mild thinning of bone mass) and *osteoporosis* (a loss of normal bone density that leads to fragile bones and an increased risk of bone fracture). People who are on carbamazepine often have slight increases in liver enzymes measured on blood tests; these are not harmful. However, higher elevations, or elevations that continue to rise, may be a sign of liver injury.
▶ Drug–drug interactions:
  ▷ Antifungal agents, cimetidine, diltiazem, erythromycin, clarithromycin, fluoxetine, omeprazole, propoxyphene, and verapamil can increase carbamazepine levels, causing toxicity. Antipsychotics, antifungal agents, cyclosporine, felbamate, lamotrigine, narcotics, neuromuscular blockers, oral contraceptives, theophylline, tiagabine, topiramate, tricyclic antidepressants, valproic acid, and warfarin can be affected by carbamazepine, causing a decrease in their effectiveness.
  ▷ Carbamazepine can lower the effectiveness of oral contraceptives (birth control pills).

Ethosuximide (Zarontin)

▶ Used for absence (*petit mal*) seizures.
▶ Common side effects:
  ▷ Gastrointestinal distress, drowsiness, irritability, sleep disturbances, or dizziness.
▶ Rare side effects:
  ▷ Skin rash, blood disorders, psychosis.
▶ Drug–drug interactions:
  ▷ Carbamazepine, phenobarbital, and phenytoin may lower ethosuximide levels.

Felbamate (Felbatol)

▶ Felbamate is used for partial seizures, and for the generalized tonic–clonic seizures, typical and atypical absence, and atonic and myoclonic seizures associated with the Lennox-Gastaut syndrome.
▶ Common side effects:
  ▷ May cause *anorexia* (loss of appetite), nausea, insomnia, headache, dizziness, fatigue, weight loss, double vision, and unsteadiness.
▶ Rare side effects:
  ▷ After using felbamate on more than 100,000 patients, 32 cases of life-threatening bone marrow failure and 10 cases of hepatic failure were reported, some resulting in death.

The use of felbamate is usually restricted to people with difficult-to-control epilepsy, and written consent is required prior to use. Frequent laboratory testing will be required, usually weekly to monthly during the first year of treatment, then every 3 months thereafter.

▶ Drug–drug interactions:
  ▷ Phenytoin, carbamazepine, and phenobarbital can decrease felbamate levels. Valproic acid can increase felbamate levels. Felbamate can increase phenobarbital, phenytoin, valproic acid, and carbamazepine epoxide levels, and can lower carbamazepine levels.

Gabapentin (Neurontin)

▶ Used for partial seizures. Contraindicated in absence seizures and other generalized epilepsies.
▶ Common side effects:
  ▷ Sedation, fatigue, unsteadiness.
▶ Rare side effects:
  ▷ Leg swelling.
▶ Drug–drug interactions:
  ▷ None reported.

Lacosamide (Vimpat)

▶ Lacosamide is indicated for partial seizures, including simple partial, complex partial, and secondarily generalized tonic-clonic seizures.
▶ Common side effects:
  ▷ May cause double vision, dizziness, headache, and nausea.
▶ Rare side effects:
  ▷ None have currently been identified, but lacosamide has only been used in a small population to date, and some very rare side effects (occurring in less than 1/1000 people) may not yet have been identified.
▶ Drug–drug interactions:
  ▷ None have been identified.

Lamotrigine (Lamictal)

▶ Used for partial seizures, and for primary generalized tonic-clonic, typical and atypical absence, and atonic and myoclonic seizures associated with the Lennox-Gastaut syndrome.
▶ Common side effects:
  ▷ Dizziness or unsteadiness, headache, insomnia, double or blurred vision, nausea, or drowsiness.
▶ Rare side effects:
  ▷ Up to10% of people who take lamotrigine will develop a skin rash or other sign of allergic reaction, such as swollen lymph glands or fever. If the drug is continued, a small per-

centage will progress to *Stevens-Johnson syndrome*, which is a potentially fatal condition. The incidence of rash may be higher in children, when the drug is combined with valproic acid, with a high initial dose, or when the dose is increased too rapidly. If a rash occurs, the drug must usually be stopped without delay.

▶ Drug–drug interactions:

▷ Oxcarbazepine, phenytoin, carbamazepine, phenobarbital, and primidone can lower lamotrigine levels. Valproic acid will increase lamotrigine levels. Lamotrigine will increase valproic acid levels by approximately 25%. Oral contraceptives will lower lamotrigine levels. Pregnancy will lower lamotrigine levels.

Levetiracetam (Keppra, Keppra XR)

▶ Used for partial and generalized tonic–clonic seizures, myoclonus, and absence.

▶ Common side effects:

▷ Irritability, dizziness, difficulty with balance or coordination, sleepiness, nausea, abdominal pain, tremor, headache.

▶ Rare side effects:

▷ None reported; the dose should be adjusted for elderly people or people with kidney disease.

▶ Drug–drug interactions:

▷ None reported.

Oxcarbazepine (Trileptal)

▶ Used for partial seizures, generalized tonic-clonic seizures. May worsen absence (petit mal) or myoclonic seizures.

▶ Common side effects:

▷ Sedation, dizziness, difficulty with balance and coordination, double vision or abnormal vision, nausea, gastrointestinal distress, or tremor.

▶ Rare side effects:

▷ Oxcarbazepine can reduce the body's ability to regulate water and salt balance, causing an abnormality in the sodium level; this is called *hyponatremia*. Symptoms of hyponatremia may include nausea, tiredness, headache, sedation, or confusion. People with an allergy to carbamazepine have a 25% to 30% chance of being allergic to oxcarbazepine.

▶ Drug–drug interactions:

▷ Carbamazepine, phenobarbital, phenytoin, and verapamil can lower the effectiveness of oxcarbazepine. Oxcarbazepine can lower the effectiveness of felodipine, lamotrigine, and oral contraceptives. Oxcarbazepine can increase phenytoin levels.

Phenobarbital

▶ Used for partial seizures, generalized tonic–clonic seizures; it may also be used for absence and myoclonus.
▶ Common side effects:
  ▷ Sedation, dizziness, difficulty with concentration, irritability, and mood changes, such as depression. Children may become hyperactive.
▶ Rare side effects:
  ▷ Allergic reaction, *hepatotoxicity* (liver problems), and blood disorders; symptoms could include rash, fever, enlarged lymph nodes, unusual bleeding or bruising, severe stomach pain, nausea and vomiting, or a change in skin color.
▶ Potential long-term effects:
  ▷ Osteopenia or osteoporosis, *Dupuytren's contractures* (painless thickening of the deep tissue that passes from the palm into fingers), and frozen shoulder. Phenobarbital may lower sexual *libido* (sexual desire).
▶ Drug–drug interactions:
  ▷ Felbamate and valproic acid can increase phenobarbital levels. Phenytoin may increase or decrease phenobarbital levels. Phenobarbital can decrease the effectiveness of antipsychotics, carbamazepine, cyclosporine, felbamate, griseofulvin, itraconazole, ketoconazole, lamotrigine, narcotics, oral contraceptives, phenytoin, steroids, tiagabine, theophylline, topiramate, tricyclics, valproic acid, and warfarin.

Phenytoin (Dilantin, Phenytek)

▶ Used for partial seizures, generalized tonic–clonic seizures.
▶ Common side effects:
  ▷ Double or blurred vision, headache, dizziness, unsteadiness, and drowsiness. Bleeding, tenderness, or swelling of the gums may occur, which may be prevented by good oral hygiene including brushing, flossing, gum massage with a toothbrush, and regular visits with the dentist. Unusual hair growth on the body and face may occur.
▶ Rare side effects:
  ▷ Allergic reaction, hepatotoxicity (liver disease), bone marrow depression (failure of the bone marrow to produce sufficient blood cells), *systemic lupus erythematosus* (a chronic autoimmune inflammatory disease), and *lymphadenopathy* (abnormally enlarged lymph nodes). Symptoms seen could include rash, fever, enlarged lymph nodes, unusual bleeding or bruising, severe stomach pain, nausea and vomiting, change in stool color, or a change in skin color.

▶ Potential long-term effects:
  ▷ Osteopenia or osteoporosis, *peripheral neuropathy*, *folate deficiency*, and *cerebellar atrophy*.
▶ Drug–drug interactions:
  ▷ Amiodarone, cimetidine, diltiazem, felbamate, fluconazole, fluoxetine, isoniazid, omeprazole, oxcarbazepine, phenobarbital, ticlopidine, and topiramate can increase phenytoin levels. Antacids, carbamazepine, ciprofloxacin, phenobarbital, and sucralfate can lower phenytoin levels. Phenytoin can lower the effectiveness of antipsychotics, azole antifungal agents, carbamazepine, cyclosporine, felbamate, lamotrigine, narcotics, neuromuscular blockers, oral contraceptives, steroids, tiagabine, theophylline, topiramate, tricyclics, valproic acid, and warfarin.

Pregabalin (Lyrica)

▶ Used for partial seizures and generalized tonic–clonic seizures.
▶ Common side effects:
  ▷ Drowsiness, dizziness, unsteadiness, blurred vision, trouble concentrating, dry mouth, weight gain, and swelling of the feet, legs, or hands.
▶ Rare side effects:
  ▷ Skin rash; muscle pain, soreness, or weakness.
▶ Drug–drug interactions:
  ▷ None known.

Primidone (Mysoline)

▶ Indicated for partial seizures and primary generalized tonic–clonic seizures.
▶ Common side effects:
  ▷ Similar to phenobarbital.
▶ Rare side effects:
  ▷ Similar to phenobarbital.
▶ Drug–drug interactions:
  ▷ Primidone is converted to two active metabolites, phenobarbital and phenylethylmalonamide. Phenytoin and carbamazepine will decrease primidone levels but increase phenobarbital levels. Isoniazid and nicotinamide will increase primidone levels and decrease phenobarbital levels. (See phenobarbital for other drug–drug interactions.)

Rufinamide (Banzel)

▶ Rufinamide is demonstrated to be effective for seizures associated with the Lennox-Gastaut Syndrome, as well as partial seizures.

▶ Common side effects:
  ▷ May case headache, dizziness, fatigue, somnolence, unsteadiness, double vision, and nausea.
▶ Rare side effects:
  ▷ None have currently been identified, but rufinamide has only been used in a small population to date, and some very rare side effects (occurring in less than 1/1000 people) may not yet have been indentified.
▶ Drug–drug interactions:
  ▷ Rufinamide may increase phenytoin levels by 20%. Valproate may increase rufinamide levels, especially in children, by up to 70%. Phenytoin, phenobarital, and carbamazepine can decrease rufinamide concentrations by 30%. Rufinamide may slightly reduce carbamazepine and lamotrigine levels.

Tiagabine (Gabitril)

▶ Used for partial seizures and generalized tonic–clonic convulsions.
▶ Common side effects:
  ▷ Dizziness, lack of energy, drowsiness, difficulty concentrating, confusion, weakness, gastrointestinal distress, nervousness, irritability, tremor, and insomnia.
▶ Rare side effects:
  ▷ Spike-wave stupor.
▶ Drug–drug interactions:
  ▷ Carbamazepine, phenytoin, and phenobarbital can lower tiagabine levels. Tiagabine can lower valproic acid levels by 10%.

Topiramate (Topamax)

▶ Used for partial seizures; generalized tonic–clonic seizures; atonic, tonic, and tonic–clonic seizures in Lennox-Gastaut syndrome; can be used for myoclonic and absence seizures.
▶ Common side effects:
  ▷ Difficulty concentrating, drowsiness, nervousness and anxiety, slowed speech, depression, decreased appetite and weight loss, numbness or tingling of the hands or feet, tremor, nausea, and vomiting.
▶ Rare side effects:
  ▷ There is an increased risk of developing kidney stones, so adequate fluid intake must be maintained. Diamox and Daranide should be avoided, as these medications in combination with topiramate can contribute to kidney stone formation. *Glaucoma*, with symptoms of blurred vision or eye pain, is possible. Decreased sweating, which can lead rarely to heat stroke in children, has been reported, as has *metabolic acidosis*.

▶ Drug–drug interactions:
  ▷ Phenytoin, carbamazepine, and phenobarbital can lower topiramate levels. Topiramate can increase phenytoin levels by 25%. Topiramate can lower the effectiveness of oral contraceptives.

Valproic Acid (Depakote, Depakene)

▶ Used for partial seizures; primary generalized tonic–clonic, typical and atypical absence, atonic, myoclonic seizures.
▶ Common side effects:
  ▷ Nausea, vomiting, drowsiness, difficulty concentrating, dizziness, hair thinning, and weight gain.
▶ Rare side effects:
  ▷ Hepatotoxicity (liver disease), *pancreatitis* (inflammation of the pancreas) *thrombocytopenia* (decreased amount of platelets in the blood), bone marrow failure; symptoms could include rash, fever, enlarged lymph nodes, unusual bleeding or bruising, severe stomach pain, nausea and vomiting, or a change in skin color or color of stool.
▶ Potential long-term effects:
  ▷ If taken for many years, valproic acid can be associated with cysts in the ovaries, which may lead to irregular periods and problems with fertility.
▶ Drug–drug interactions:
  ▷ Felbamate and fluoxetine can increase valproic acid levels. Carbamazepine, lamotrigine, phenobarbital, and phenytoin can lower valproic acid levels. Valproic acid can increase the levels of carbamazepine epoxides, felbamate, lamotrigine, phenobarbital, free phenytoin, and zidovudine.

Zonisamide (Zonegran)

▶ Used for partial seizures; generalized tonic–clonic seizures, tonic, and myoclonic seizures.
▶ Common side effects:
  ▷ Dizziness, difficulty with balance, fatigue, loss of appetite, nausea, headache, and tremor.
▶ Rare side effects:
  ▷ There is an increased risk of developing kidney stones, so adequate fluid intake must be maintained. Decreased sweating, which can lead rarely to heat stroke in children, has been reported.
▶ Drug–drug interactions:
  ▷ Carbamazepine, phenobarbital, and phenytoin can lower zonisamide levels. Grapefruit juice can lower zonisamide levels.

MEDICATIONS LESS OFTEN USED

Other medications may be chosen by your doctor. These drugs are the best choice for some people, but they are not as frequently used as those described earlier.

Acetazolamide (Diamox)

▶ This is a mild *diuretic* (increases urination) that has some antiseizure effect. It is often prescribed to women who typically have seizures just before their menstrual periods. This medication can be used for 1 week, prior to menses, or on an everyday basis. Its effectiveness may wear off if used on a daily basis.

▶ Common side effects:
  ▷ Numbness of the hands or feet, loss of appetite, nausea, diarrhea, and increased urination. Potassium loss may occur, which may be indicated by muscle cramps and unusual tiredness or weakness. You may want to drink extra orange juice or eat a banana daily to increase your potassium intake.

▶ Rare side effects:
  ▷ Allergic reaction. People who are allergic to sulfa medications may be allergic to acetazolamide.

Ethotoin (Peganone)

▶ Indicated for partial seizures and generalized tonic–clonic seizures.

▶ Common side effects:
  ▷ Nausea, vomiting, *nystagmus* (constant, involuntary eye movements), and dizziness. Should be taken with meals to reduce the incidence of gastrointestinal distress.

▶ Rare side effects:
  ▷ Allergic reactions, hepatotoxicity (liver disease), blood disorders, and lymphadenopathy (disease of the lymph nodes). Symptoms could include rash, fever, enlarged lymph nodes, unusual bleeding or bruising, severe stomach pain, nausea and vomiting, or a change in skin or stool color.

▶ Drug–drug interactions:
  ▷ Unknown, but may be similar to phenytoin.

Mephobarbital (Mebaral)

▶ Indicated for partial seizures and primary generalized tonic–clonic seizures.

▶ Common side effects:
  ▷ Same as phenobarbital and primidone.

▶ Rare side effects:
  ▷ Same as phenobarbital and primidone.

▶ Drug–drug interactions:
  ▷ Same as phenobarbital.

Methsuximide (Celontin)

▶ Indicated for typical and atypical absence seizures.
▶ Common side effects:
  ▷ Gastrointestinal distress, drowsiness, headache, dizziness, hiccups, irritability, and behavioral changes.
▶ Rare side effects:
  ▷ Allergic reactions and blood disorders.
▶ Drug–drug interactions:
  ▷ Phenytoin, carbamazepine, and felbamate can increase methsuximide metabolite levels. Methsuximide can increase phenobarbital, phenytoin, and carbamazepine metabolite levels. Methsuximide can lower carbamazepine levels.

BENZODIAZEPINES

Benzodiazepines are a large group of chemically similar *psychotropic drugs* (medications that effect behavior) that include diazepam (Valium), rectal diazepam (Diastat), lorazepam (Ativan), clonazepam (Klonopin), clorazepate (Tranxene), alprazolam (Xanax), clobazam (Frisium), and several other brands. They are most often prescribed as mild tranquilizers but have some important uses for seizures.

The most important use of benzodiazepines is for *emergency treatment*. Because these drugs can be given *intravenously* (through a vein) and therefore work within a few minutes, they are commonly used in emergency rooms and hospitals to stop seizures quickly. Some are also available for home use, by mouth, rectal suppository, or nasal spray, to stop severe or recurring seizures.

These medications are also used daily to prevent seizures for some people, but they have three disadvantages: they tend to make people sleepy, the anti-seizure effect may wear off in a few months, and, if they are stopped suddenly, severe seizures may result. Those benzodiazepines most commonly used for epilepsy are discussed here. Other side effects may include depression, trouble thinking clearly, and slowed reaction times.

Diazepam (Valium, Diastat)

Diazepam is given intravenously to stop seizures quickly, but the effect wears off in a few minutes, so that additional doses or another medication must be added soon. Oral Valium is rarely used for seizures because of sleepiness. Diastat is a diazepam gel in a prefilled tube; it is given in the rectum to stop repetitive seizures. It causes sleepiness but is very safe and is designed to be used only occasionally. It is an excellent choice for people who tend to have "clusters" of seizures; that is, who are likely to have more than one seizure in a day. It can be used at home, and may prevent the need to go to an emergency room.

Lorazepam (Ativan)

This is the first choice of many doctors for use in emergency situations to stop seizures. When given intravenously, it usually stops seizures within a few minutes. Unlike diazepam, the effect lasts several hours. It can be used by mouth at home for this purpose, but by mouth it takes at least 30 minutes to have an effect.

Clonazepam (Klonopin)

Clonazepam is sometimes useful, especially for absence seizures or myoclonic seizures. If it is stopped suddenly, dangerous seizures may occur.

Clorazepate (Tranxene)

When taken by mouth, this medication lasts longer than some of the other benzodiazepines, and is sometimes used for complex partial seizures and other seizure types.

Clobazam (Frisium)

Not available in the United States, but prescribed in Canada and other countries, this medication may have less tendency to lose its effect with time than some of the other benzodiazepines.

BROMIDES

Bromides are bitter, salty-tasting liquids containing bromide. Bromide is interesting from a historical standpoint because it was the first medication that really worked well to control seizures. It was therefore the first real AED. It was discovered by an English physician in 1857, and was the most commonly used drug for seizures until phenobarbital was discovered in 1912. Bromides are rarely used now because they usually cause drowsiness and acne. However, for a few people, they are very effective. Bromides have to be made up specially by a pharmacist; they are not commercially available.

FREQUENTLY ASKED QUESTIONS

Q How does my doctor choose a medication to treat my seizures?

A Prior to embarking on potentially long-term antiepileptic medication therapy, a diagnosis of epilepsy must be made. This diagnosis is based on several factors, such as history, a physical and neurologic examination, and diagnostic testing. From this information, your doctor will try to determine what type of epilepsy you have. A medication will then be selected based on seizure type, the presence of other illnesses and medications, the cost of the drug, how the drug must be dosed (one, two, three, or four times a day), and the potential side effects. Once a medication is selected, the dose will be adjusted at various intervals. Your doctor will try to use one medication, and she will increase the dose until your seizures are controlled or you develop side effects. It may be necessary to try several medications before finding one that causes no side effects and controls your seizures. There may be times when multiple medications will need to be used together.

Q Do all antiepileptic medications cause side effects?

A All medications, not just seizure medications, have the potential of causing mild or severe side effects. Many people start a medication and experience no side effects at all, or only mild side effects that are easily resolved by adjusting a dose. As with any medication, more serious side effects can occur and must be addressed immediately.

Q Will I need to take seizure medication forever?

A The decision to withdraw medication is never an easy one. Your doctor must take into account the likelihood of seizure recurrence off medication, the risks of injury with seizure recurrence, and the risk of potential long-term drug effects. Some types of epilepsy require life-long treatment; *juvenile myoclonic epilepsy* is a genetic form of epilepsy that rarely goes away. Other children, however, may experience a benign form of epilepsy that they outgrow.

Q Can I take the generic form of seizure medication?

A Generic formulations may not be appropriate with some of the antiepileptic medications, because of the difference in the bioavailability of the drug (the amount of medication actually absorbed by the body). Generics are allowed a 20% difference in bioavailability. If a generic medication is needed because of financial concerns, the same generic company should be used with each refill. If a person switches from a name-brand to generic drug, toxicity or seizure recurrence is a possibility.

Q What do I do if I can't afford the medication?

A Financial concerns should be discussed with your doctor, prior to starting a new medication. Your doctor may be able to assist you with obtaining the medication you need. Generally, older medications are not as costly as some of the newer seizure medications, and many times these can be just as effective as the newer medications. Most pharmaceutical companies participate in patient-assistance programs, which are programs that supply the patient with medication, free of cost, if they meet financial eligibility requirements. Sometimes, a change in the pill size is all that is needed to make a medication affordable. Frequently, there is little difference between the costs of various pill sizes. For example, instead of using a 100-mg pill twice each day, change the pill size to 200 mg and take half a pill twice a day. Simple things, such as using mail order pharmacies over local pharmacies, may save you money.

My Notes

_____

_____

_____

_____

_____

_____

_____

5

EPILEPSY SURGERY

Indications and Procedures

Key Points

▶ Epilepsy surgery is safe and effective in selected patients with intractable epilepsy.

▶ Surgery should be considered by anyone whose seizures are not completely controlled by medication.

▶ Epilepsy is, in some people, a serious and potentially life-threatening illness.

▶ The purpose of surgical evaluation is to identify a single, abnormal part of the brain that is epileptic and can be safely removed.

▶ After preoperative tests are completed, the neurologist should review all test results with you, and then ask you to meet with a neurosurgeon.

▶ Seizure outcome depends on the specific epilepsy syndrome, the type of pathology causing the epilepsy, the surgical procedure used, and other factors.

Epilepsy surgery is not new or experimental. It has been around for over 100 years. In fact, the first few operations were performed by pioneering surgeons during the late 1800s. Once neurosurgery became safer, epilepsy surgery was reborn again in the 1940s. Epilepsy surgery is now performed at many centers in the United States and abroad, and many thousands of patients have been operated with good outcome. In this chapter, we describe the indications, procedures, testing, and outcome related to epilepsy surgery.

REASONS FOR EPILEPSY SURGERY

The goal of medical or antiepileptic drug (AED) therapy is to prevent all seizures from occurring. Should that not be possible, then AEDs are used to minimize the severity and reduce the frequency of seizures as much as possible, to enable people with epilepsy to lead as normal a life as possible. The goal of surgical therapy is no different, because it aims at the same target.

When should someone consider having surgery as a treatment for epilepsy? Surgery should be considered by anyone whose seizures are not completely controlled by medication—that is, when seizures continue to occur despite properly taking appropriate anticonvulsant drugs. In this circumstance, surgery often offers a relatively safe and effective means of either completely stopping seizures, or at least reducing their severity or lessening their frequency. In practice, surgery is a reasonable option only if stopping or reducing seizures would improve a patient's quality of life or reduce his risk of injury or death from recurring seizures.

Surgery may seem a drastic step for symptoms that rarely occur in some patients, especially when many individuals are able to carve out happy and fulfilling lives for themselves despite having epilepsy. However, uncontrolled epilepsy can cause many problems, some mild and others quite serious, and these can appear at any time, often long after epilepsy has begun. These complications may be medical or psychosocial, and will be discussed later in this book. Surgery is considered precisely because it is effective in treating some forms of epilepsy, and the risks of surgery are often lower than the long-term risks of uncontrolled seizures.

People come to an epilepsy center for a variety of reasons. Often, they are unhappy either with the seizure control provided by their current treatment or with the unacceptable side effects of their AEDs. Some patients come to get a more precise diagnosis. Whatever the reason, when first arriving at an epilepsy center, you should not be surprised if your physician discusses brain surgery with you. This is because many epilepsy specialists want to inform patients about all their possible treatment options when they begin to care for them. A doctor may describe treatments that are appropriate now, some that may be needed in the future, and other that may ultimately never be recommended.

Many patients coming to an epilepsy specialist for the first time have already thought about surgery. Some have misconceptions. As a result, they are afraid to discuss surgery or become upset if the doctor brings it up. Nevertheless, most people appreciate an honest discussion about surgery.

WHO IS A CANDIDATE FOR SURGERY?

What kinds of seizures and types of epilepsy lead people to consider having surgery? Seizures that lead people to consider surgery are usually those that cause alterations of awareness (consciousness), since these have the potential to produce injury and disrupt the quality of life. Most commonly, people who have surgery have either *complex partial* or *secondarily generalized tonic–clonic* (*grand mal*) seizures (see Chapters 1 and 2). These seizures, by virtue of interrupting consciousness, have adverse psychosocial and medical repercussions. Loss of awareness prevents the legal operation of a motor vehicle, forces people to rely on others for transport, limits independence, reduces employment opportunities, reduces educational choices, and imposes psychological burdens. Simple acts, such as riding a public bus, are burdened in ways that people who have not experienced seizures cannot imagine. In addition, if seizures cause someone to precipitately fall to the ground (for example, tonic–clonic seizures or *drop attacks*), then serious injury might occur. Lastly, some seizures, although they might not cause falling or loss of awareness, might be so unpleasant or upsetting that surgery could still be an option. For example, a seizure that periodically gives rise to intense nausea and vomiting, or one that leads to socially unacceptable behavior, might warrant consideration of surgical therapy. In general, the individual who suffers from the seizures is the only one who can state with certainty whether the residual symptoms are inadequately controlled and might warrant surgical treatment.

How often should seizures occur to consider surgery? There is no scientifically determined seizure frequency required to consider surgery. While most people who have surgery have seizures at least once per month, others have had fewer seizures and decided that surgery was worthwhile. After all, having just one or two seizures per year prevents someone from driving and can have serious medical and psychosocial consequences. Some patients may have only a few seizures per year, but these episodes are severe and serious every time they occur. In our experience, some patients with as few as two or three seizures per year have had surgery and viewed it as worthwhile. Careful preoperative counseling should always be done so that patients will have realistic expectations.

When the seizures occur might also influence the decision to have surgery. Seizures that occur at predictable times pose fewer problems than erratically occurring seizures. For example, a person who has seizures occurring only while asleep (*nocturnal seizures*) may drive an automobile and live a relatively unrestricted life. However, it should be noted that these seizures might still be psychologically disturbing to the patient and his family, and still may pose a risk for injury or death. Unfortunately, most patients have seizures that occur in an unpredictable way.

Last, the type of epilepsy influences the decision to consider surgery. Some types of epilepsy are known to disappear with the passage of time; it would be overly aggressive to perform surgery for a condition that will remit in the near future. Other types of epilepsy are believed to have a progressive downhill course (for example, *progressive myoclonic epilepsy*), so that surgery will certainly not afford long-term benefit and should not be done. Other types of epilepsy (for example, *medial temporal lobe epilepsy*) are known to be resistant to medical therapy and do not remit; these often respond favorably to surgical treatment, so surgery might therefore be offered in those conditions.

RISKS OF EPILEPSY

In this section, we will review the risks posed by epilepsy. Not every complication occurs in all people; the severity of the problems varies from person to person, and some fortunate individuals may live full lives without difficulty. Scientists do not completely understand why and how many of these complications happen, but the simple fact remains that epilepsy is, for some people, a serious and potentially life-threatening illness. The adverse consequences of epilepsy can occur in people with mild seizures as well as severe seizures, and it is impossible to predict when they might occur.

By and large, complications occur in people who have uncontrolled seizures. People whose epilepsy is completely under control—that is, people who are not having any seizures—have little to fear from their condition. However, ongoing seizures (*recurrent seizures*) often pose risk, which depends on the type of seizure and the rate at which they occur. The major determinants are: severity of seizures, how often they occur, whether consciousness is altered, whether seizures cause falling, whether they produce psychologically or physically unpleasant symptoms, and whether they cause socially unacceptable or embarrassing behavior (e.g., disrobing, incontinence).

The medical risks can be placed into one of several broad categories: bodily injury, brain injury, and death.

Seizures can cause direct bodily injury, such as lacerations, bruises, fractures, burns, and internal injury. For example, if a seizure causes a person to fall, he might fracture a bone in the fall or suffer a laceration of the skin. If the seizure happens while driving a motor vehicle, a more serious injury might occur, not only affecting the driver, but possibly affecting other occupants of the car and innocent bystanders who might not even be in that vehicle.

Brain injury arises for two reasons. First, seizures may cause brain damage due to the excessive release of certain chemicals within the brain. In addition, some seizures, especially tonic–clonic (*grand mal*) lead to lower levels of oxygen in the blood, which can also cause brain injury. Seizures may place stresses on other parts of the body and it is not uncommon to find heart damage in people with epilepsy who have uncontrolled tonic–clonic seizures. Lastly, people with uncontrolled seizures are at greater risk for dying than people whose seizures are controlled. The reasons for this are uncertain, but it is known that perhaps half of these excess deaths are sudden and unexplained, and the other half are from ordinary causes including pneumonia, heart disease, and cancer. The sudden unexplained deaths are believed to be caused by either *respiratory arrest* (stopping breathing) or heart rhythm abnormalities that are provoked by seizures or occur in the aftermath of a seizure. Evidence suggests that the risk of death in people who have successful surgery (with complete seizure control after surgery) becomes lower, reverting back to that of the general population.

The psychosocial risks of uncontrolled epilepsy are manifold. People are more apt to experience depression, anxiety, and other psychological problems when seizures occur on a frequent basis. This may be due to several factors, including changes in the way the neurons in the brain communicate with one another, changes in brain chemistry, and for behavioral reasons (e.g., losing a job because of a seizure would make anyone unhappy). Socially, people with uncontrolled seizures experience a variety of difficulties because of their seizures. The degree of educational attainment is often lower, and occupational opportunities are more limited. When children have seizures, parents tend to be overprotective (a natural response), which can alter psychological development and restrict independence. Inability to drive limits independence as well in the modern world, with resulting restrictions on social activities and employment. People with uncontrolled seizures are less likely to marry, and they earn less money than people whose seizures are controlled. Evidence suggests that surgery can reverse some of these detrimental effects if their seizures are stopped. After successful surgery, patients are most likely to socialize and change marital status, earn more money, drive a vehicle, and engage in a wider range of social activities than people who continue to experience uncontrolled seizures.

PRESURGICAL EVALUATION

Once it is decided that surgery is to be considered, patients will undergo outpatient and inpatient testing (see the next sections). This may be quite time-consuming and may spread out over several months. Time must be scheduled away from home or work to complete the testing. Family or friends may also need to take time off to accompany patients to the testing and to provide care at home after testing is complete. Many epilepsy centers expect patients to set aside at least 1 week, and to be ready to take part or all of a second week for monitoring by video and electroencephalogram (EEG) with scalp electrodes; this is known as *video-EEG* (V-EEG) monitoring. If intracranial V-EEG monitoring is required, up to 6 weeks off work may be required. Patients must carefully follow the instructions given about how and when to take medications before and after V-EEG monitoring.

The purpose of this evaluation is to identify a single, abnormal part of the brain that is epileptic and can be safely removed (Table 5.1). For example, physicians might find scar tissue (a structural *lesion*) that is electrically abnormal by EEG testing in a brain area that can be safely removed. Finding a single abnormal region offers the best chance of success if one contemplates removing part of the brain to treat seizures.

TABLE 5.1
Preoperative Evaluation for Epilepsy Surgery

When done?	Always performed	Sometimes performed
Clinical information	History and examination	
Interictal EEG	Routine EEG	Electrocorticography, MEG
Neuroimaging	MRI head	FDG-PET, MRS, SISCOM, PET receptor studies
Ictal EEG	Video-EEG (extracranial)	Video-EEG (intracranial)
Cognitive evaluation	Neuropsychology	Sodium amobarbital study

History and Physical Examination

Despite all the amazing advances in medical technology, nothing surpasses the importance of the office examination. The history and physical examination are the most important tools that exist; especially the history, which provides critical information. The office evaluation helps establish what kind of seizure is present, assesses the potential causes of the seizure disorder, and helps your doctor arrive at the precise diagnosis and prognosis. After taking a history and examination, an experienced physician can usually decide whether surgery is a reasonable idea. The history and physical often contain important clues regarding the area of the brain that might be causing seizures; sometimes, a physician can even form a preliminary opinion as to the potential risks of surgery.

A doctor may begin taking a patient's history by asking about his birth and development. Any difficulties that occurred with mother's pregnancy and the patient's delivery may indicate an early insult to the brain or a congenital disorder of brain development that may result in a seizure disorder. Prematurity, infections while in the womb, brain hemorrhages, strokes, and disordered brain development may all result in epilepsy. These problems may be identified when infants and children do not meet expected milestones, such as walking and talking at appropriate ages, or after seizures appear. Any neurologic symptom, such as memory difficulty, weakness, walking difficulty, visual disturbances, and the like may provide clues to abnormal function in a particular part of the brain. This might indicate which part of the brain is producing seizures.

A detailed history about the seizures you have also provides important clues. *Auras* may indicate where seizures start, although some are not specific. For example, a seizure beginning with tingling in one hand usually starts in the opposite parietal lobe. Visual symptoms, such as flashing lights or colors, suggest that seizures originate in the occipital lobe or visual area. In contrast, déjà vu and fear often occur in temporal lobe epilepsy, but can also happen in seizures starting elsewhere, such as in the frontal lobe. The description of the movements that occur during a seizure may also help identify where seizures start. Seizures that cause lip smacking often arise in a temporal lobe while stiffening of one side might indicate the seizure has begun on the opposite side of the brain.

A physician performs a physical examination to search for signs that may help determine the diagnosis. The general examination may sometimes be as important as the neurologic examination. Analysis of vital signs like heart rate and blood pressure, skin examination, and inspection of the head, chest, and abdomen may reveal evidence of a disorder that can affect multiple organ systems, including the brain. For instance birthmarks on the skin may be characteristic of a genetic disorder like *tuberous sclerosis* or *neurofibromatosis*, disorders commonly associated with brain abnormalities and seizures. An elevated blood pressure may be a risk factor for a stroke that led to a seizure disorder.

The neurologic examination detects abnormal function of the nervous system. For example, weakness of a limb may indicate brain injury. Temporal lobe seizures are usually associated with memory impairment. Any abnormal finding may help the neurologist pinpoint the source of your seizures. However, the examination is usually normal or nonspecific, even when seizures occur frequently, and further testing is required.

Neurologic Testing

Electroencephalogram (Refer to Chapter 2)

The brain produces electrical activity that may be analyzed using an EEG machine. A routine EEG is typically collected for 30 to 60 minutes by the application of metal electrodes glued onto the scalp with a conducting paste. The electrodes are attached to wires that connect to the input box of the EEG machine. The EEG machine displays the electrical activity on a computer screen or on graph paper. For patients considering surgery, the EEG is often reviewed and the information analyzed in conjunction with all other tests (see Chapter 2 for details).

Video-EEG Monitoring (Refer to Chapter 2)

To gather more evidence for seizure localization before surgery, most physicians prefer to record and observe seizures. This is typically done in the setting of a specialized epilepsy monitoring unit in a hospital. EEG and video are recorded continuously for many days to correlate the physical manifestations of the seizure with the brain's electrical activity. Trained nurses or EEG technologists can also perform testing during the seizure. Because seizures may occur relatively infrequently in some people, antiepileptic medication doses are often reduced to induce seizures.

This reduction in dose may lead to seizures being stronger than usual, and close observation is required. Intravenous access is sometimes established when antiepileptic medications are stopped to ensure the rapid delivery of antiepileptic medication if seizures must be stopped quickly. If people fall to the ground with their seizures, restraints (such as padding, bed rails, or vests) may be used to prevent injury. People may be admitted to the hospital for a few days or up to several weeks, depending on how often their seizures occur and how many need to be studied.

Physicians usually need to study several seizures to fully ascertain their source. The EEG and video are carefully analyzed to determine which side and lobe of the brain is likely to be responsible for seizures. V-EEG monitoring can be done with ordinary electrodes glued to the scalp, or with electrodes placed directly on the brain, a process that is described in the section "Intracranial Video-EEG."

Magnetic Resonance Imaging (Refer to Chapter 2)

Nearly all patients being evaluated for epilepsy surgery require *magnetic resonance imaging* (MRI). The MRI supplies detailed anatomic information about the structure of the brain. It is highly sensitive for localizing strokes, tumors, birth defects, scar tissue from traumatic injury, and other abnormalities associated with seizures. In temporal lobe epilepsy, which is the most common type of epilepsy treated with surgery, shrinkage of a deep part of the temporal lobe (the *hippocampus*) can be seen. More sophisticated MRI techniques like *MR spectroscopy* (which images brain chemistry) and *volumetric MRI* (which measures the size of specific regions of the brain) are employed at some epilepsy centers to supplement the basic MRI information. MRI is a safe technique, although it may be uncomfortable for people who suffer from claustrophobia, because the MRI machine is a long, hollow cylinder in which the patient lies while his brain is being scanned.

Functional MRI

Functional MRI (fMRI) is useful in some people who are having epilepsy surgery. It measures changes in blood oxygen during the performance of certain tasks, such as reading, speaking, and moving, to identify which areas of the brain are responsible for those functions. By localizing these important functions, it helps guide the surgeon so that he may avoid removing parts of the brain that are necessary for critical functions.

SPECT and PET (Refer to Chapter 2)

Positron emission tomography (PET) and *single photon emission computed tomography* (SPECT) imaging tell us about the function of the brain. Both techniques use radioactive tracers that are injected into a vein. The radiation dose is very low and safe. PET measures brain metabolism when patients are not having seizures, studying how much *glucose* (a form of sugar) is used. Areas of the brain that trigger seizures typically require less energy, so less glucose is seen in that area on the scan. PET scans take approximately 75 minutes. The most common study used in the evaluation of intractable partial epilepsy is the ^{18}F-*deoxyglucose* (FDG)-PET. The disadvantages of PET include the difficulty obtaining *ictal* (during seizures) studies, the cost of the procedure, the short-lived radioactive exposure, and the limited number of scanners available. However, PET is very sensitive in patients with temporal lobe epilepsy and can aid in the decision-making process. The use of a radioactive compound precludes the performance of this study in pregnant women.

SPECT scans measure blood flow and, like PET, may be done between seizures, although they can also be used during seizures. During seizures, blood flow is selectively increased in the area that triggers seizures. The injection of radioactive tracer must take place very early in the seizure in order to reliably localize the brain region responsible. Ictal SPECT studies are more sensitive and specific than are *interictal* (between-seizures) examinations for indicating the site of seizure onset. In selected patients, ictal SPECT is very valuable for the surgical decision-making process. SPECT scans take about an hour. The disadvantage of ictal SPECT is due to the difficulty of injecting during a seizure, meaning that hospitalization and special personnel are required.

Magnetoencephalography

Magnetoencephalography (MEG) is a noninvasive, non-hazardous technology for functional brain mapping by measuring the associated magnetic fields emanating from the brain. These measurements are commonly used in both research and clinical settings. There are many uses for the MEG, including assisting surgeons in localizing a pathology, assisting researchers in determining the function of various parts of the brain, neurofeedback, and others.

The imaging technique is used to measure the magnetic fields produced by electrical activity in the brain through superconducting quantum interference devices (SQUIDs). The SQUID is a very low noise detector of magnetic fields, converting the magnetic flux into voltage allowing detection of weak neuromagnetic signals. Since the SQUID relies on physical phenomena found in superconducators it requires extremely cold temperatures for operation.

In a modern MEG device, an array of more than 300 SQUIDS is contained in a helmet shaped liquid helium containing vessel called a dewar as shown in Figure 5.1, which allows for simultaneous measurements at points all over the head. The MEG system is operated in a shielded room that minimizes interference from external magnetic disturbances such as traffic noise.

Unlike Computed Tomography (CT) and Magnetic Resonance Imaging (MRI) which provide structural/anatomical information, MEG provides functional mapping information. MRI and CT are use to map anatomy, MEG can be used to image neurological function. Using MEG, the brain can be observed "in action" rather than just viewing a still image. In addition, MEG has an extremely high temporal resolution (milliseconds) and also provides a good spatial resolution and there is no need to paste electrodes on the scalp as with EEG.

Neuropsychological Testing and the Intracarotid Amobarbital Test (Wada Test)

Neuropsychological testing consists of a complex battery of tests such as IQ tests, memory tests (both verbal and nonverbal), learning tasks, mental flexibility tasks, and an assessment of emotional and personality traits. This testing can last from 4 to 6 hours. The neuropsychologist will analyze this information to characterize cognitive and emotional function and, in some cases, to make inferences about a region of the brain that may not be working well. Sometimes this region is also the place where seizures are originating.

Before surgery, some people are referred for a *Wada* or *intracarotid amobarbital test*. This test helps identify which side of the brain is responsible for language (speech, comprehension), and

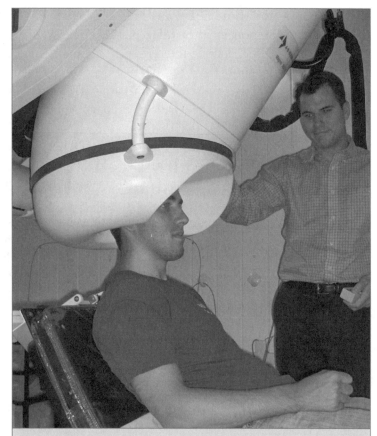

FIGURE 5.1
Patient being prepared by an assistant for a MEG scan.

assesses the memory capabilities of the temporal lobes. This test takes about 2 hours, and is done on an outpatient basis. A catheter is inserted into the femoral artery after local anesthetic is injected in the skin of the groin overlying the artery. The catheter is directed upward into the carotid artery in the neck. A short-acting sedative drug, amobarbital, is injected to temporarily anesthetize one side of the brain. Then language and memory can be assessed from the still functioning, nonanesthetized side of the brain. For example, if the left carotid artery is injected, and you cannot speak, then language is located on the left side of the brain. During the period of anesthesia (typically lasting several minutes) objects, pictures, or words may be presented to the patient. After the sedative wears off (usually about 10 minutes or so after injection), a patient can be asked to recall what was shown. In this way, memory may be assessed for each side of the brain. Knowledge of this information helps assess the risks of surgery and may confirm that a suspect temporal lobe functions abnormally. The Wada test is not necessarily required, and different epilepsy centers have different criteria for determining when it is used. It is most helpful when planning a left temporal lobectomy in a right-handed individual or if the side controlling language is uncertain and must be known.

Intracranial Video-EEG

After all the aforementioned studies are performed, the exact origin of seizures may still be uncertain in some patients. In carefully selected individuals, placing EEG electrodes directly on the surface of the brain or within the brain may help pinpoint where seizures start. These electrodes are inserted by a neurosurgeon, with the patient under general anesthesia in the operating room. *Subdural electrodes* are flat plastic strips containing EEG electrodes that are placed on the surface of the brain. Two types of subdural electrodes are used: *grids* and *strips*. Grids are rectangular plates, varying in size, but usually no bigger than 8 × 8 cm. Strips are narrower, perhaps 1 cm wide, and from 4 to 8 cm long (Figure 5.2).

Depth electrodes are inserted into sites that are situated deep within the brain. These electrodes may be placed on one or both sides of the brain, depending upon need. The wires are connected to an EEG machine after the head is carefully wrapped with a sterile dressing. V-EEG monitoring can then be performed in the same way as when electrodes are attached to the scalp. Since this is a neurosurgical procedure, it carries the same risks as any brain surgery, including bleeding, infection, stroke, and death. Chances of a permanent serious complication are small, but this possibility means that this procedure should be done only when absolutely necessary. Intracranial V-EEG recording is needed in a minority of patients, but is essential in some to determine where to operate. Paradoxically, it is sometimes safer to use intracranial electrodes

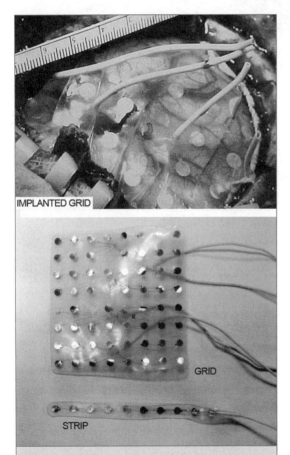

IMPLANTED GRID

GRID

STRIP

FIGURE 5.2
Surgically implanted subdural electrode grid (top). Picture of new subdural electrode grid and strip (bottom).

than to proceed directly to surgery, since better definition of the area to be removed might reduce the chances of producing a permanent neurologic complication and improve chances of success.

When electrodes are placed on the brain, they may be stimulated with a small electrical current to map brain function. For example, if a small current is applied to an electrode on top of your brain's language area, you would suddenly stop speaking until the current was turned off. If a current were applied to an elec-

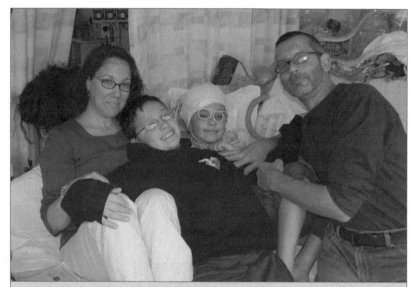

FIGURE 5.3
Patients who undergo intracranial VEEG monitoring are able to move comfortably and interact normally with those around them such as family members.

trode lying over the motor region of your hand, your hand muscles might contract or twitch. By mapping these areas, the surgeon can then avoid removing them during surgical removal of the epileptic brain region.

Intracranial V-EEG monitoring can take as little as several days or as long as several weeks. Depending on individual circumstances, surgery might be performed immediately upon concluding the monitoring, or electrodes might be removed and surgery scheduled several weeks later (Figure 5.3).

SURGICAL PROCEDURES

Three types of operations are offered to treat epilepsy. Most commonly, the part of the brain responsible for producing seizures is removed. This is called *resective surgery* and includes *focal cortical resection*, *anterior temporal lobectomy*, and *hemispherectomy*. If seizures come from a single place that cannot be safely removed, then a procedure called *subpial transection* is done, in which small parallel cuts are placed in the offending brain region; this too may alleviate seizures. Last, when multiple areas of the brain cause seizures, a disconnection procedure called *corpus calloso-*

tomy (or anterior corpus callosotomy) might be performed. This is a *palliative* procedure, used to reduce the number of seizures and their severity, although it does not completely eliminate seizures.

Surgical Discussion

After preoperative tests are completed, the neurologist should review all test results with you, and then ask you to meet with a neurosurgeon. This is also a time to review the test results and clearly understand the chance of benefit and the risks of a complication or undesired outcome with surgery. Patients should compare those chances against the likelihood of benefit and the risk of problems if they continue with nonsurgical treatments. They should also review with the surgeon all the medications taken, discuss any problems they have had with anesthesia or previous operations, and tell the surgeon about any other serious medical problems they may have. For example, patients often ask how long it will take to recover and how much personal assistance they will need from others once they get home.

Doctors often prefer that you bring along the person who will care for you at home after surgery. This allows your caregiver to hear and help you remember the discussion. This person should also ask questions.

After discussing the risks, goals, rationale, and alternatives associated with the surgery, you or your legally authorized representative will be required to sign a form stating that you have been informed about and understand these issues and consent to undergo the surgery. After signing an *informed consent* form, patients must make certain that they follow the preoperative instructions exactly as instructed. Some of these instructions may include where and when to report on the day of surgery, when to get certain blood tests, what medications to avoid before surgery (for example, aspirin and ibuprofen), what to do if another illness arises, what to bring to the hospital, or what to leave home. Usually patients are asked not to eat anything after midnight the day before surgery, although medications can usually be taken with a sip of water on the day of surgery.

Surgical Procedures

Focal Cortical Resection

When a localized (*focal*) area of the brain is found to cause seizures, it may be possible to remove this area and eliminate the seizures, however, this area of brain must be dispensable. In other words, the tissue to be removed should not be one of the critical brain areas (*cortex*) that are required for movement, sensation, language, or vision. Removal of these important areas can lead to permanent impairments. Fortunately, other brain functions such as personality, intelligence, and the senses of taste and hearing are spread over large areas of cortex. As a result, small focal cortical resections are not likely to cause major deficits in those brain functions.

Focal cortical resections often involve brain surface areas that are found, through testing, to contain physically abnormal tissue. Abnormalities can include scar tissue, benign or malignant tumors, blood vessel malformations, congenital brain malformations, and other abnormalities. MRI and other imaging techniques may not find a visible *anatomic abnormality*; in these situations, EEG recordings, PET scans, and fMRI are used to show the area of brain *functional abnormality*. The surgery often ideally is planned to remove the entire anatomic lesion, the functionally abnormal cortex, or both. However, the presence of nearby critical brain areas, blood vessels, and numerous other factors may limit the size of the resection that can be safely performed.

Anteromedial Temporal Resection or Anterior Temporal Lobectomy

For patients with epilepsy in whom seizures appear to arise in the deep part (*medial area*) of the temporal lobe, partial removal of the temporal lobe is performed. In this case, a removal of the front (*anterior*) portion of the temporal lobe is often the first step of the surgery. This part is similar to a focal cortical resection. This may be done in a standard fashion under general anesthesia or while awake. In this surgery, the surgeon may remove the lobe to a certain distance back from the tip. A direct recording of the electrical activity of the brain cortex (an *electrocorticogram* or ECoG) may also be performed. Some surgeons prefer to perform this step when the patient has been awakened from light general anesthesia so that many different areas of the exposed brain cortex can be stimulated with low electrical currents. This is done to find areas that might be important for language. In that case, the surgeon will remove the cortex from the tip back as far as he can, without removing language areas. Either way, the next step is for the surgeon to remove the inner (medial) area of the lobe that contains deeper brain structures known as the *hippocampus* and part of the *amygdala*. Some surgeons remove these medial tissues as a whole unit, and others remove them piece-by-piece (Figure 5.4).

Memory is the main brain function supported by the temporal lobe. Indeed, many patients with temporal lobe epilepsy have problems with their verbal or visual-spatial short-term memory before surgery. At a few epilepsy centers, surgeons may prefer to primarily remove the medial structures. This variation of medial temporal lobe surgery is called an amygdalohippocampectomy, and is often a more difficult surgery to perform. It may be done on the belief that it might minimize the chance of memory impairment that can occur with temporal lobe resections. However, many studies suggest that several things predict a low risk of substantial worsening of memory with temporal lobe resections. These include visible abnormal tissue in the hippocampus on MRI, onset of epilepsy as a young child, and surgery on the side of the brain opposite to the one in which language function is mainly located. Specifically, in most right-handed people, language is localized to the left hemisphere of the brain, so that right temporal lobe surgeries seldom significantly worsen language and verbal memory abilities. As a result, AMTR is more commonly performed than amygdalohippocampectomy.

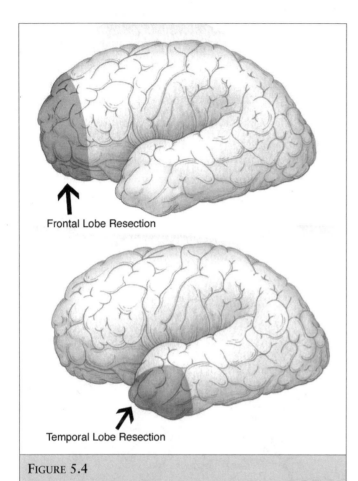

FIGURE 5.4
Rendering showing the approximate areas removed during (shaded areas) standard frontal lobectomy (right top) and temporal lobectomy (right bottom). (Modified from Orrin Devinsky, MD, NYU)

After AMTR, some patients will lose a small portion of their upper visual field on the side opposite from surgery. This is usually unnoticeable by the patient. Visual testing may reveal that the patient is not able to see objects well in the upper quadrant of their peripheral vision on the side opposite the surgery. This does not pose a problem for people who want to drive after surgery.

Corpus Callosotomy

The *corpus callosum* is a very large bundle of white matter that connects the right and left hemispheres of the brain. *White matter* is made up of very long, thin, tube-like extensions of brain cells (*axons*) surrounded by an insulating material (*myelin*). When brain cells (*neurons*) make electrical signals, axons move the signals over long distances where they can then interact with a second group of neurons. This is how the brain transmits signals, or communicates, across distances. In generalized epilepsies, long axons connecting the left and right sides of the brain allow epileptic electrical discharges to rapidly spread throughout the brain.

Corpus callosotomy was first performed in 1939 to treat epilepsy. It was based on the observation of a patient whose generalized seizures improved as a tumor involving the corpus callosum grew larger. There was little interest in callosotomy until the 1960s, when a neurosurgeon published findings on the clinical and neuropsychological outcome of the surgery. Since then, many corpus callosotomies have been performed, and the technique has been improved to reduce neurologic problems after surgery. The technique now involves an initial incision in the scalp at the top of the head. The surgeon then separates the two hemispheres of the brain. Looking into the fissure between the two hemispheres, the surgeon can see the corpus callosum. In patients who do not have severe neurologic handicaps, the structure is then cut beginning at the front end, and often extending 75% to 90% toward the back end. Usually, the entire callosum is not cut in order to minimize neurologic disconnection syndromes such as inability to read, left arm and leg clumsiness resembling weakness, and inability to name things felt only with the left hand. In some patients with severe preexisting disabilities such as severe mental retardation and inability to read, the entire corpus callosum may be cut (Figure 5.5).

Corpus callosotomy is often used when other treatments have failed to reduce the number of seizures in patients with severe generalized epilepsies with neurologic impairments due to a variety of conditions. Callosotomy can reduce, but almost never completely eliminate, seizures that cause sudden loss of muscle strength and falls (*atonic seizures*). It may also reduce the number of generalized tonic–clonic seizures (*convulsions*) and seizures causing sudden body stiffening (*tonic seizures*).

After callosotomy, patients usually recover overnight in an intensive care unit. Right after surgery, fever can occur, seizure frequency may increase, temporary left-sided weakness may be present, and patients may temporarily talk less. With newer techniques, leg weakness and bladder incontinence are less common compared to the past.

Multiple Subpial Transection

The most effective surgical treatment for partial seizures is a removal (resection) of part of the brain. As mentioned earlier, this cannot be performed if the seizure focus lies within indispensable cortex. For this reason, the technique of *multiple subpial transections* (MST) was developed. Some of the underlying conditions for which MST has been used are Landau-*Kleffner syndrome*, *Rasmussen syndrome*, scars, and birth malformations of brain cortex (Figure 5.6).

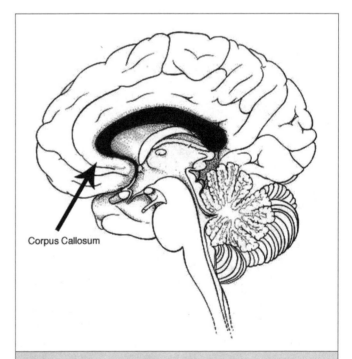

Corpus Callosum

FIGURE 5.5
Midline view of the brain showing the corpus callosum (black shaded) area which is sectioned during a corpus callosotomy.

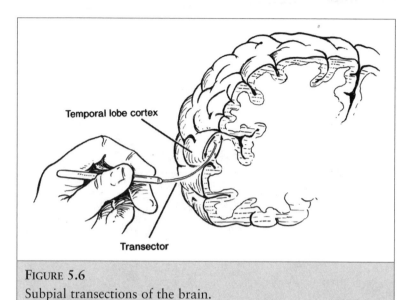

Temporal lobe cortex

Transector

FIGURE 5.6
Subpial transections of the brain.

The technique was first described in a large group of patients in 1989. Since then, many physicians have reported good reduction of seizures with little or no neurologic deficits using MST. The procedure involves placing surgical cuts parallel to each other through the cortex, perpendicular to the long axis of an out-folding (*gyrus*) of the brain. MST can be performed as the sole surgical procedure, or it can be accompanied by focal cortical resection. How MST reduces the number of seizures is not fully known, but is thought to be related to cross-cutting of nerve fibers that run horizontally across the cortex, thereby limiting the spread of electrical seizure discharges.

Patients who undergo MST must understand that this procedure reduces the number of seizures but usually does not completely eliminate them. Some patients can have new or worsened neurologic problems after MST, but these are usually only mild and temporary. These temporary problems are usually related to the area of cortex that undergoes MST.

Hemispherectomy

A small percentage of persons have seizures that arise from a large area of only one *hemisphere* (one-half) of the brain. This is usually related to a physical condition in one hemisphere of the brain that is present since the time of birth or early childhood. Examples of brain disorders causing medically refractory seizures are birth malformations of the cortex, strokes occurring before or just after birth, tuberous sclerosis, and Rasmussen syndrome. Patients who are candidates for hemispherectomy typically have significant weakness on the opposite side of the body (*hemiparesis*). Generally, the more severe the hemiparesis, the less likely patients will have significant worsening of the weakness after surgery (Figure 5.7).

In the past, the offending hemisphere was simply removed surgically. However, this sometimes led to long-term complications in which repeated low-level bleeding developed in the remaining brain structures. Therefore, the surgery performed today is known as a modified, or *functional hemispherectomy*. This involves separating the upper lobes of the hemisphere from the deep (central) core of the brain and from the opposite hemisphere. This upper separated hemisphere is left in place, connected to its blood vessels, but all the white matter bundles passing up and down on that side, and the corpus callosum, are severed.

Vagus Nerve Stimulation

Vagus nerve stimulation (VNS) is designed to treat seizures by sending mild pulses of electrical energy to the brain through the vagus nerve. Experimental work showed that long-term

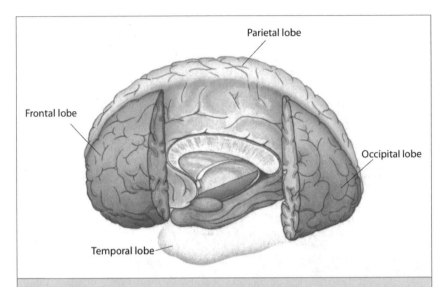

FIGURE 5.7
Side view of the left hemisphere, showing the area of brain removed (*light shaded*) and the areas of brain disconnected from the opposite hemisphere (*dark shading*) in a hemispherectomy. (Courtesy of Orrin Devinsky, MD, NYU)

stimulation of the vagus nerve in animals and humans can reduce the frequency of seizures. The vagus nerve itself is a part of the autonomic nervous system, which controls bodily functions that are not under conscious control such as heartbeat, breathing, and sweating. How exactly the VNS helps with seizures is not known.

The VNS is the only FDA approved electrical stimulation treatment for seizures. The device has been implanted in over 25,000 patients worldwide including many children.

The major indications for VNS are:

▶ Patients with intractable seizures who are not candidates for brain surgery.
▶ Patients who have failed brain surgery for epilepsy

All potential patients should undergo testing as those patients undergoing brain surgery. The device consists of two parts; a generator (similar to a pacemaker) and a connecting wire. During surgery, two incisions are made, one for the implantation of the device and the second to wind the wire form the stimulator around the vagus nerve on the left side of the neck. The process generally is completed in 1 or 2 hours and the brain is not involved during the surgery (Figure 5.8).

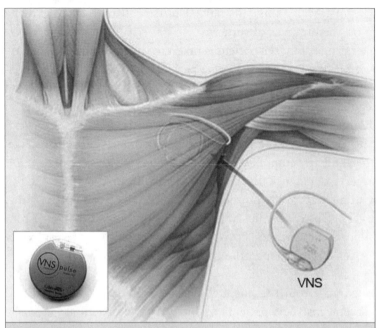

FIGURE 5.8
Image showing an actual VNS device (lower left) and the location where the VNS is implanted.

Stimulation is produced by a small generator which is implanted under the skin below the left collar bone. The device is flat and round like a silver dollar, 4 cm wide and 10 to 13 millimeters thick, depending on the model used. Newer models may be somewhat smaller.

The generator sends impulses from the vagus nerve in the neck to the brain and delivers therapy in two ways. A doctor can program a 24-hour a day, seven-day a week "dose" of intermittent stimulation. One dosage frequently used is 30 seconds of stimulation followed by a five-minute period of no stimulation. The stimulation is automatically delivered. The second use of the device is when a patient or family member senses a seizure coming on (an aura), they can pass a magnet over the area in the chest where the generator is implanted activating extra simulation to suppress the seizure. In some patients, this may stop a seizure.

The battery for the stimulator lasts approximately 5 to 10 years. Although the surgery is relatively safe, a small number of patients may have vagus nerve injury that can result in voice changes and hoarseness. In addition, some patients may cough or have difficulty talking while the stimulator is on.

The VNS has been shown to improve seizure control in about 30-40% of patients. Significant seizure reductions are seen in about 25% of patients while very few become seizure free.

POSTSURGICAL RECOVERY

Most operations for epilepsy take 4 to 6 hours. Before entering the operating room, the patient goes to a preanesthesia area to meet the anesthesiologist and see the neurosurgeon. From there, the patient is taken to the operating room, where he is moved onto the operating table. After anesthesia is started, the operation begins. Many surgeons have a nurse call the family midway during the operation to update them on the progress of surgery.

Immediately after leaving the operating room, the patient is taken to the postanesthesia recovery area for a few hours. After recovering from anesthesia, some patients are taken to in an intensive care unit for close observation until the next day or longer. After that, patients are transferred to an intermediate care units or a regular hospital ward with other neurologic and neurosurgical patients, until they are ready to go home.

The length of time spent in the hospital depends a lot on the type of surgery, side effects, age, the presence of other medical problems, and any complications from surgery. Pain is the most common symptom that occurs after surgery, but it usually becomes relatively mild within 3 days. Nausea and vomiting may occur within the first 24 hours, and occasionally for a longer time. Sometimes, a seizure occurs after surgery. This can be upsetting, but studies suggest that a postoperative seizure does not necessarily indicate that your epilepsy will continue. This may be especially true if it occurs right after surgery. After a typical operation, many patients can be discharged 3 days after surgery.

When epilepsy patients are discharged from the hospital, they usually feel quite tired and complain of head pain. The neurosurgeon instructs patients about activity restrictions, when he should be seen, and what kinds of symptoms and signs need to be reported right away. Some things that should be reported are fever, worsened headache, vomiting, seizures, scalp swelling, and leakage of fluid or blood from the incision.

After returning home, the rate at which patients return to normal activities again depends on type of surgery and individual age, level of general health and fitness, and pain tolerance. After focal cortical resections or anteromedial temporal resections, most patients can walk well within the first week after surgery; require some assistance with feeding, bathing, or dressing for 2 to 3 weeks; can resume part-time work with no lifting after about 4 weeks; and can return to full-time light duty work at 6 weeks after surgery. Many surgeons advise avoiding lifting or exertion for 6 weeks.

SEIZURE OUTCOME AFTER EPILEPSY SURGERY

Surgery can result in complete seizure control, reduction in number of seizures, decreased seizure intensity or duration, or no benefit. Rarely, some patients may experience worsened seizure control after surgery. Seizure outcome depends on the specific epilepsy syndrome, the type of pathology causing the epilepsy, the surgical procedure used, and other factors. (In this section, when an approximate percentage for seizure freedom is given, it applies to those groups of patients treated with that surgery who, for the most part, continue to take at least one medication for seizure control.)

In general, the most effective procedure is a focal resection of small benign tumors. Most reports in the scientific literature estimate a 90% chance of seizure freedom 1 year after this particular type of surgery. The procedure with the next highest seizure-free rate is anteromedial temporal resection (AMTR) or anterior temporal lobectomy. When this surgery is done in patients who have an early risk factor (febrile seizure as an infant or toddler) or when a detailed brain MRI scan shows scarring in the hippocampus of the medial temporal lobe, the seizure-free rate 1 year later is approximately 65% to 80%. A recent review of the scientific literature found that only one-quarter of adults and one-third of children have discontinued medication and remain seizure-free 5 years after AMTR. Most patients who are seizure-free choose to remain on at least one drug for many years. This may be because about half of patients who are seizure-free on drugs after surgery will have a seizure recurrence if they stop all medication. When AMTR is performed in patients with no early childhood risk factor, adult age of onset, or completely normal temporal lobes on MRI scan, then the seizure-free rate is roughly 50%. Some recent studies have found evidence that the seizure-free rate measured 1 year after surgery declines slightly when again measured at 5- and 10-year time intervals after AMTR. The seizure-free rates cited here refer to current seizure status—that is, the proportion of patients who have been seizure-free for at least 1 or 2 years when last examined. The proportion of patients who never have another seizure after surgery may be as low as 40% to 50% once 10 years have passed since surgery, and some patients may still experience auras although complex partial seizures have stopped.

After focal cortical resections in frontal, parietal, or occipital lobes in which no physical abnormality is seen on MRI, about 50% or less of patients stop having seizures. For resections in these areas when lesions such as birth malformations of the cortex, blood vessel malformations, old strokes, or other scar tissue are present, the seizure-free rate depends on how completely the abnormal tissue can be safely removed and how large or widespread the pathologic tissue area. For brains that have more than one damaged area (for example with traumatic brain injury or infections), the seizure-free outcome may be much less than 50%. Physicians must give patients the best estimate of the likelihood of seizure-freedom, which must be individualized.

With corpus callosotomy, some 70% to 80% of patients experience a decrease in seizure numbers by at least half their previous rate. Certain types of seizures may be reduced at higher rates, including tonic, atonic (drop attacks), and tonic–clonic (grand mal) seizures. Complex partial, myoclonic, and atypical absence seizures are often not helped by corpus callosotomy.

As mentioned earlier, MST is considered to be a treatment to reduce, but not to eliminate seizures. A research study in 2001 that gathered data from many different American epilepsy centers reported that two-thirds of patients had a worthwhile reduction in complex partial seizures. Seizures may return in perhaps 20% of cases. Complete seizure freedom is rare. Seizure-free results can be better for Landau-Kleffner syndrome, and many of these children show improved language development. The results for Rasmussen syndrome, however, are poorer because of the progressive nature of the disorder. Seizure-free rates may be as high as 90% for hemispherectomy in children with epileptic areas confined to the hemisphere being treated with surgery.

OPERATIVE COMPLICATIONS

With any surgery, there is a risk of bleeding or infection. The chances of these are minimized in various ways, and usually there is about a 1% to 2% risk of each of these complications. Infections are nearly always successfully treated with antibiotics, and most bleeding does not cause significant problems. On occasion, however, bleeding can be life-threatening. When the skull and the coverings of the brain (*meninges*) are opened to allow for the operation, a small chance exists that the cerebrospinal fluid surrounding the brain can leak out and collect under the scalp. This can be treated in a few ways, but sometimes requires repeat surgery to stop the leak. A small and uncertain percentage of patients experience persistent headaches that occasionally are hard to treat. This can occur in persons with a long history of a headache disorder, or it can occur for the first time.

During surgery, nearby critical brain areas could be damaged either directly if a clot develops in a blood vessel or if bleeding occurs. The chance of these occurrences depends on the type of operation and other factors. If the resection involves the anteromedial temporal lobe, then special complications may occur. These include difficulties with naming and with memory. In most right-handed persons, there may be language problems and problems remembering verbal material after a left-sided AMTR. After right-sided AMTR, there may be difficulty remembering visuospatial or other nonverbal material, but this is usually only detected with sophisticated neuropsychological testing and is rarely apparent to patients. In left-handed or ambidextrous persons, language can be located in either hemisphere, and right-sided surgery could cause naming or verbal memory difficulty.

Psychiatric disturbances may follow AMTR. This has not been researched extensively, but research suggests that depression is probably the most common psychiatric problem after surgery. It may occur more often in people with a history of depression before surgery, but can be seen in people with no history of depression. It typically occurs 2 to 6 weeks after surgery, and improves within a few months. In a small number of patients, anxiety or *psychosis* (unusual thinking) can occur after surgery. This occurs more commonly in people with a history of these problems before surgery. Although these symptoms usually respond to medication, at times they can be difficult to treat.

After surgery that renders patients seizure-free, close relationships and marriages may experience strain. This happens because patients feel better and are more energetic and independent. This changes relationships, especially ones in which the patient has been very dependent on the spouse. Often this is temporary, but occasionally it can produce long-lasting problems in the relationship. Conversely, many relationships improve. The improvement in energy level fosters better interactions with the spouse, stronger sexual drive, and less depression over the long run.

Immediately after corpus callosotomy, some patients experience fever or temporary leg weakness. Depending on the amount of corpus callosum that is sectioned and the degree of developmental disability of the patient, there may be some permanent signs of a disconnection syndrome after surgery. This can be seen in various ways, but can include difficulty following commands to perform tasks using one arm (usually the left), not using that arm as much as the other, unintentionally doing different things with one hand or leg, and difficulty reading.

After MST, neurologic problems occur in about 20% of patients. The vast majority of the time, these are temporary and, if permanent, are mild.

After hemispherectomy, marked weakness and complete loss of vision on the side opposite surgery will result if the patient has good use of the hand, fingers, or foot, or has good vision. However, often, there is moderately good recovery of strength in the leg. This usually means that the patient can walk fairly well after hemispherectomy, although he may not perform fine movements with the toes and foot.

Future Directions

Local Brain Stimulation

In the United States, research studies are under way to look at a device that delivers electrical current to a brain area that triggers seizures, in an attempt to shut down the seizure. These devices use electrodes that have been inserted directly on the brain surface and that are attached to a computer and stimulator. When a seizure occurs, the device recognizes it and gives an electrical stimulus. Whether this technique will work, and how effective it will be is unknown at present.

Deep Brain Stimulation

Deep brain stimulation was used in the early 1970s to control epilepsy, and it has been used for almost 10 years to treat Parkinson disease and essential tremor. It is now being studied with epilepsy again. It involves placing electrodes into the various areas of the brain and delivering intermittent electrical stimulation, whether seizures occur or not. Stimulation may help prevent seizures, perhaps both in partial and in generalized epilepsies.

Stereotactic Radiosurgery

Stereotactic radiosurgery is not really surgery in the traditional sense. The procedure involves administering beams of radiation from outside the skull, at various angles, which are all aimed at the same small target deep in the brain. The objective is to use radiation to destroy epileptic tissue instead of doing an operation to remove it. This treatment is being tested to see if it is effective and whether it can replace surgery in some partial (focal) epilepsy syndromes.

CONCLUSION

Epilepsy surgery is a good treatment choice for many people. It is a reasonably safe and effective therapy when medications do not completely control seizures. Surgery is underutilized because of lack of knowledge on the part of patients and physicians. It is important to recognize that the consequences of uncontrolled epilepsy can be dire, and that seizures might not be inevitable. Surgery affords properly selected patients a good chance of achieving seizure control, thereby helping them gain independence and improve their quality of life. People should discuss this option with their physicians or with an epilepsy specialist when seizures are not controlled by medication.

FREQUENTLY ASKED QUESTIONS

Q What types of epilepsy respond best to surgery?

A Several types of epilepsy respond well to surgical treatment. Medial temporal lobe epilepsy, in which seizures emanate from the deep part of the temporal lobe called the hippocampus or amygdala, is often successfully treated by surgery. Surgery is also usually successful when seizures come from an obvious lesion that is seen in the MRI, provided the EEG also shows an epileptic abnormality in the same area. Lastly, drop attacks, known as atonic or tonic seizures, also respond nicely to surgery.

Q What types of presurgical testing are performed to determine if I am a candidate for surgery?

A The medical history is the most important part of the evaluation process. The physician obtains information regarding the seizure symptoms, type of seizure, seizure frequency, background neurological history, and details of medical treatment. The testing that is performed serves to confirm the diagnosis made by the physician. The tests aim to find a structural lesion in the brain, show that the lesion is epileptic, and must be consistent with the background historical information. MRI and EEG are the tests that usually provide the most information. However, other tests can help establish whether surgery is possible, including PET scanning, SPECT scanning, MEG, the Wada test, and neuropsychological testing.

Q Will I be able to quit taking my antiepileptic medications after I have surgery?

A Physicians typically advise that patients continue to take their medications for a period of time after surgery. Opinions differ regarding the length of therapy after surgery. Some recommend as little as one year, while others advise remaining on medication indefinitely. Most advise continuing medication for 2 to 5 years. Medication doses are often reduced sooner, upon physician discretion.

Q Can surgery eliminate all my seizures?

A Surgery eliminates all seizures in some people, but many continue to experience some seizures after surgery. Your doctor can estimate the chances of complete seizure relief for you. This depends on the type of epilepsy, the type of operation, and other factors. Even when seizures are not completely stopped, most patients experience a major reduction in the number of seizures that they have.

Q What are some of the side effects I might have after surgery?

A The side effects depend upon the type of operation that is being contemplated and your present neurological state. The most common operation, anterior temporal lobectomy, has the potential to adversely affect memory, mainly when done on the side of the brain that controls speech. However, the chances of a serious, disabling memory decline after surgery is relatively small, and some of the preoperative tests can predict who is at greatest risk. Also, a small, usually insignificant visual field loss can occur that does not usually cause symptoms or cause disability. Operations in other lobes of the brain have the potential to compromise language abilities or cause weakness, impairment of sensation, or partial loss of vision. Since operations in these areas are individualized, no general statements can be made and patients should discuss specific risks with their physicians. In general, however, efforts are made to minimize the chance of causing a permanent neurological deficit, since the goal of surgery is to make life better, not worse.

My Notes

_____

_____

_____

_____

_____

6

DIET AND ALTERNATIVE THERAPIES FOR EPILEPSY

Ketogenic Diet, Herbs, and Supplements

Key Points

▶ Ketogenic diet is useful as a treatment of seizures. Most patients treated with the ketogenic diet are children.

▶ The ketogenic diet is effective with more than 30% to 40% of people on the diet having more than 90% improvement in their seizure control.

▶ Possible side effects in association with the diet, include a heart disorder, pancreatitis, vitamin and mineral deficiencies, anemia, reflux, bruising.

▶ Herbs and Chinese medicine are widely used with standard drugs. However, no scientific study has shown beneficial effects of these therapies.

▶ Melatonin can be of help in the management of sleep disorders and epilepsy in some patients.

▶ All alternative methods for seizure treatment should be discussed with your doctor before you start.

YOU SHOULD KNOW THAT DIETARY CONTROL of disease is not a new idea. A perspective on how this has evolved may help you understand why this therapy is useful, and may be helpful as you pursue optimizing your care with your doctor. Throughout antiquity, civilizations recognized that fasting and other forms of dietary manipulation could lead to improved health. These beliefs clearly influenced biblical tradition. Rafael's *The Transfiguration* shows Jesus casting out the devil, and disciples report that Jesus said it was done by prayer and fasting (Matthew 17:14–21). These methods continued to be referenced in religious works, but did not find their way into science and modern medicine until the 20th century.

KETOGENIC DIET

Mythology has always surrounded epilepsy, including the belief that seizures were caused by dietary excesses. But out of this mythology has come an important therapy for seizure control. In the 19th century, the French reported improvement in seizures using programs of fasting. This technique was subsequently tried in New York, in a program created by Hugh Conklin, a doctor of osteopathy. Conklin was a disciple of the pioneering physical cultist, Bernarr Macfadden, who advocated diet to cure disease. Conklin put his patients on a "water diet"—a strict, very-low-calorie diet—to cure seizures. One particular child, the nephew of John Howland, Professor of Pediatrics at Johns Hopkins, was cured of very severe epilepsy by this fasting and water diet. Rawle Geylin adapted the diet, and used it successfully with a number of other patients. Impressed by the results, the child's father, John Howland, provided funds for the diet to be studied. Thus, during the first decades of the 20th century, investigators finally had the tools to begin to unravel the metabolic mysteries of nutrition.

Fasting leads to a condition called ketosis, which is described in detail in the next section. In 1921, R. M. Wilder of the Mayo Clinic was the first to propose an actual diet that would mimic the biochemical effects of fasting. It was high in fats (ketogenic foods) and low in carbohydrates and protein (antiketogenic foods). This diet, modified in various ways over the ensuing decades, still forms the basis of ketogenic diet therapy.

The use of the diet decreased during the latter half of the 20th century because of the introduction of phenytoin and other important anticonvulsant medications. (It always seems easier to take a pill than to change a lifestyle.) However, the diet resurfaced during the 1990s, with publicity from the Charlie Foundation. The Foundation was started by Jim and Nancy Abrahams, parents of Charlie Abrahams, who was cured of severe intractable epilepsy while on the diet. Today, the ketogenic diet is being adapted and used worldwide as an important tool in seizure therapy.

How the Diet Works

Exactly how the ketogenic diet works is unknown. Doctors know that fasting and the ketogenic diet clearly change the way in which the body uses energy. During fasting, *ketone bodies* (chemicals like acetoacetate, B-hydroxybutyrate, and acetone) are formed in the blood. These chemicals become the brain's source of energy, rather than it's usual source, which is *glucose* (a kind of sugar that the body derives from the digestion of carbohydrates).

Scientists think that it's possible that the ketone bodies themselves, particularly acetone, may have anticonvulsant properties. In addition, the ketogenic diet may alter *neurotransmitters*, the chemicals that transmit electrical energy within the brain. The diet also may change energy metabolism in the brain or simply provide less energy to the brain so that it won't support seizures. Because the ketogenic diet is very low on carbohydrates (similar to the popular Atkins' weight-loss diet, it provides the brain with a very stable and somewhat low level of glucose that may also be important in the control of seizures. Because the diet is high in fats, an excess of important *lipids* (fats) in the bloodstream might also have a direct effect on the brain.

During the last decade, there has been a substantial increase in the basic science surrounding the ketogenic diet, and someday we may actually understand why it works. If this happens, it may be possible to provide a therapy that is less restrictive than the present diet.

How Well Does the Ketogenic Diet Work?

Should you consider using the ketogenic diet? It worked in the 1930s, and it still works today. But, because it requires a lot of commitment from you, your family, and your epilepsy treatment team, you must understand how likely it is to be of benefit before investing the time and effort required in doing it.

Most patients treated with the ketogenic diet have been children. Early studies reported that 40% to 60% of children on the diet had more than a 90% improvement in seizure control. Even studies in the 1990s, in epilepsy cases where very modern drugs had been used and failed, reported that almost 30% of patients had virtually complete seizure control while on the diet. When a large number of studies are surveyed, it appears that 30% to 40% of people on the ketogenic diet have more than 90% improvement in their seizure control, and another 30% have a 50% to 90% improvement.

The diet is not an easy program to stick with. The largest *prospective study* showed that about 50% of the children who start the diet actually remain on it at 1 year, largely because it has been effective in their controlling seizures. Of those who stayed on the diet for 1 year, 7% were seizure free, 20% had more than a 90% reduction in their seizures, and 23% had a 50% to 90% decrease in seizures.

Children and the Ketogenic Diet

Some children should not be put on the diet, including those with special *metabolic disorders* like pyruvate carboxylase deficiency, most mitochondrial disorders, and fatty acid oxidation problems. On the other hand, some metabolic disorders, like glucose transporter deficiency and pyruvate dehydrogenase deficiency, use the ketogenic diet as a critically important therapy.

Although the cause for seizures is not found in most children with epilepsy, you should be sure that your child has had an appropriate work-up before using the diet. It's important that the doctor and the dietician who will be designing your child's diet know of any metabolic problems that would make the diet dangerous.

Most seizure types respond to the diet. However, some studies suggest that partial or focal seizures might not be as well controlled. (If your child's seizures are not well controlled, and they are coming from one part of the brain [focal seizures], it is important to know if your child is a good candidate for surgery. If surgery is appropriate, this has a much better chance for a cure than using the diet.) The diet may be a very useful therapy in some of the myoclonic seizure disorders of early childhood, as well as in tuberous sclerosis and infantile spasms.

Age also doesn't appear to be a critical factor, and many adolescents have been successfully treated with the diet. Success for an adolescent is improved when he is an active participant in food choice, and when the diet is sensitive to his physical as well as social needs. Teenagers need food that doesn't make them feel "different" from their peers. They need to have a positive attitude about choosing those foods that will allow them to have control over their seizures. (The diet has not been used or studied extensively in adults.)

Starting the Ketogenic Diet

This is not a do-it-yourself cure for epilepsy! In the wrong hands, the diet could be very dangerous. The ketogenic diet should be administered by a team trained and experienced in its use. This team must include, at a minimum, a physician and a dietician with knowledge of the intricacies of administering the diet. The physician should be experienced in working with the diet, monitoring its side effects, and manipulating the diet in collaboration with a dietician. The keto team must be in place before beginning the program.

If you are going to a center that has little experience with the keto diet, ask if that center has access to support from one with much more experience—a big brother or sister in the field. There is no such thing as a "certified" center, but you should only do the diet with people who have a wide range of experience in using this therapy.

The ketogenic diet can be started in various ways. Some centers call for hospitalizing the child for 4 days, during which time the child fasts for 24 to 48 hours. Then, gradually, the diet is introduced over the next 3 days. Other centers may begin the diet without fasting, or start the diet on an outpatient basis. Hospitalization allows for careful observation of the child to see how she responds to fasting, a very controlled application of the diet, and a thorough education of the family.

Family education is very important. The keto education program includes extensive information about the diet, how to calculate and prepare meals, how to monitor the child, how to respond when the child is ill, and how to observe for side effects. You may want to know how fasting will affect your child, because sometimes a brief fast is used when a child has been on the diet but is having *breakthrough seizures*. A brief fast may sometimes return a child to good seizure control. Knowing what to expect makes the diet safer and easier to do.

In preparation for placing your child on the diet, the nutritionist will review her dietary history, allergies, food preferences, and nutritional status. You may be asked to recall what (and how much) your child has eaten for the last 3 days. In general, the youngest children are placed on a 3:1 ratio diet. That means that the child is given 3 grams of fat for every 1 gram of combined protein and carbohydrate. Older children are routinely started on a 4:1 ratio diet (4 grams of fat to 1 gram protein/carbohydrate). These ratios translate into calories: every 4 grams of fat accounts for 36 calories, while 1 gram of protein/carbohydrate accounts for 4 calories. These 40 calories are considered 1 *dietary unit*. The number of calories that will be prescribed is in the range of 75% to 85% of the recommended daily allowance for your child. The dietician will often make a decision to start your child on the number of calories she is reported to be consuming at home prior to the diet, based upon your current 3-day dietary history. This is particularly true if your child is close to her ideal body weight. Otherwise, calories are restricted or added, depending on the intake needed to have your child approach ideal body weight.

As an example, let's consider that a 15-kg child might require 68 calories (kcal), per kilogram (kg) of body weight, per day. This would amount to a diet of 1,000 calories per day. If this child were placed on a 1,000 calorie diet at a 4:1 ratio, she would require 1,000 ÷ 40, or 25 dietary units. Remember that a dietary unit on a 4:1 ratio has 40 calories in it. The child would need a meal plan that included 25 × 4 = 100 grams of fat. Each day, 900 calories would come from fats, because each gram of fat has 9 calories. The other 100 calories would be from proteins and carbohydrates. A child should eat about 1 gram of protein per kilogram of body weight each day to stay healthy and provide for reasonable growth, so 15 grams of this diet should be consumed as protein. The other 10 grams are then allotted to carbohydrates. That's not much starch or sugar!

Once these calculations are complete, the dietician then creates several meal plans and menus to provide this formulation. It's important that you communicate clearly what your child will, and won't, eat. It's interesting to know that some early studies show that children with seizures actually seem to choose foods that are high in fat instead of high-carb foods, like candy. Parents are often surprised to find that their children really almost crave high-fat foods. Something in the child may be telling her that foods high in carbohydrates make her feel bad.

Meal plans usually provide three meals and one snack. With creativity, and the help of good computer programs that can readily calculate the dietary units your child must have, appetizing meal plans can be created. For example, a day's meals for a 1,000-calorie, 4:1 ratio diet for our hypothetical 15-kg child might be the following:

▶ Breakfast: Quiche with bacon; water or a diet soda
▶ Lunch: Salad with avocado, pineapple, and pecans; water or a diet soda

▶ Dinner: German sausage with potato and sauerkraut; creamy milkshake for dessert
▶ Snack: Cheesecake with blueberries

Children on the keto diet also need to consume at least 80% of the recommended daily requirement of fluids, to prevent problems like constipation and kidney stones. Most children must be coaxed to consume even this amount, so parents need to be creative. Fun foods like snow cones, popsicles, and Jell-O are great ways to get the fluids in.

The diet can be started in many ways, but the classical approach uses an initial fast. When the diet is introduced during hospitalization, fasting can be hard on families—it's usually harder on parents than it is on the child, who often sleeps a great deal during this time. Sometimes children become very ketotic and begin to vomit. They may actually need small amounts of sugar (as apple juice) to ease the situation.

After the fasting period is over, children usually receive one-third of their first ketogenic calculated meal at dinnertime of the second hospital day. This is routinely given as eggnog since this seems more palatable than tiny amounts of "real food" such as pats of butter or tablespoonfuls of cream. On day 3, breakfast, lunch, and dinner are still eggnog: one-sixth of the day's calories are given for breakfast, one-sixth for lunch, and two-thirds for dinner. On day 4, breakfast and lunch are still eggnog at one-sixth of the day's calories each, but dinner comes as a ketogenic meal that supplies the remaining two-thirds of calories. Children are routinely discharged after a breakfast of full calories on day 5, with prescriptions for a sugar-free vitamin and mineral supplement, as well as an additional calcium supplement.

Very young children and even children who are fed by gastrostomy tubes can be given the ketogenic diet. It is actually quite easy to convert a child who is taking regular formula to a ketogenic formula using special products that do not contain sugars. The dietician can provide a formula that uses a product like Ross Carbohydrate-free (protein) along with Microlipid or other oils (fats) and a carbohydrate such as Polycose. Children with gastrostomy tubes can use a similar formula. The only time when this becomes a problem is when children have significant absorption problems; these children may not be candidates for the diet.

During diet initiation, families are intensively taught to understand the framework of the diet and how to prepare the prescribed meals. Foods are actually weighed on electronic scales so that measurements are accurate to about 1 gram. Fluids are measured in cubic centimeters. Some families also use a computer program that allows them to calculate a wider variety of individualized meals so that the diet can be adapted to the fluctuating needs of their child and her family. For example, if a family is planning to visit grandparents for dinner, it's easy to call ahead and find out what is being served, then calculate a new meal for the child based on the food that will be available at Grandma's house.

Families are also taught about the various medical issues that are magnified by being on the diet. This includes constipation, caring for the child during illness, and monitoring for kidney stones. Constipation is a serious issue for many children on the diet, because the keto diet is seriously lacking in fruits and vegetables. To prevent constipation, the diet can be tailored to include *medium-chain triglycerides* (MCTs) or perhaps corn oil, or digestive agents such as MiraLax and aloe vera may be added. It's also very important to get your child to drink plenty of liquids as well.

A very important part of initiating the diet is learning how to care for your child during illnesses that involve vomiting and diarrhea, which are more problematic for children on the diet since every calorie and every drop of fluid counts! You must be sensitive to the increased need for fluids and electrolytes during this time. One way to do this is to monitor how often your child is urinating. Clear fluids like diet ginger ale may be helpful, but if your child is not able to keep down the fats that make up the major portion of her diet, she will not have enough calories available for energy needs. At times like this, you may need to use diluted portions of Pedialyte or Gatorade before you can resume the routine diet. You should understand how to do this before you go home on the diet, but you should probably be in touch with your pediatrician if your child becomes sick and you need to use these techniques.

Kidney stones are of some concern. You must learn how to observe for signs such as blood-tinged urine, pain on urination, and even nonspecific or *referred pain*. If you notice blood in the urine, a *urinalysis* is done to determine if there is really blood in the urine. If there is, your child will be sent for ultrasound to determine if stones are present, and a renal specialist should be consulted. Your doctor will try to prevent this situation by establishing whether your child is at increased risk of stones by measuring the ratio of calcium to creatinine in her urine. This is easy to do, and should be done before your child starts the diet and routinely during follow-up. If this ratio is higher than 0.2, your child should be put on Polycitra, which is a powder that is dissolved in liquid and given three times a day.

You will also need to learn how to monitor ketosis. This involves routinely checking the urine for ketones using a *urine dipstick*. A dipstick is a little piece of paper that you dip in or dampen with urine. After a few seconds, it changes color to indicate the level of ketones present in the urine. Children should show 3+ to 4+ urine ketones, particularly in the afternoon. It isn't unusual to see lower urine ketones in the morning. If this is associated with increased seizures in the morning as well, your child may need more food in the evening, so that more ketones are made to protect her from seizures through the night and into the next day.

Monitoring and Maintaining the Diet

Once the diet has been initiated, you need to maintain contact with the team via phone and e-mail. It's a good idea to keep a seizure calendar to monitor the impact of the diet on seizure frequency. Heights and weights from your child's pediatrician can provide information about the impact of the diet on growth and nutrition. If your child is gaining or losing weight, the dietician will re-evaluate the meal plans, first being sure that you are actually following the diet that they have prescribed. Sometimes communication problems crop up, or errors are made in weighing or measuring, and the dietician needs to be certain that instructions are clear. If it's necessary, calories are adjusted according to your child's actual needs. If your child continues to have seizures, the team will reconsider both the ratio and the calories. Although most people would presume that the diet wasn't working because a child was eating too much, that is frequently not true. A child must have sufficient nutrition to actually provide enough energy to make the ketone bodies. Sometimes a child really needs more food, not less. And, sometimes, children do better on lower ratios, rather than higher ratios. Because no one really understands the exact way in which the keto diet affects seizures, each child's diet must be individualized to work properly.

Children return to their clinic for follow-up on a routine basis, usually at 3, 6, and 12 months. Very young babies, or children who are medically very fragile, are often seen more frequently. During these visits, the team verifies that your child is healthy, reviews the seizure situation, discusses issues related to the diet, and provides appropriate support and changes to the diet as needed. At these visits, the team also determines whether medications can be discontinued, since it's known that the majority of children on the diet can be weaned successfully from some, and perhaps all of their anticonvulsant medications.

The team also reviews blood work, especially the *lipid profiles*, to evaluate whether alterations in sources of lipids should be changed. For example, if cholesterol or triglycerides are particularly high, your child may need meal plans that have less saturated fats. Your child may need more MCTs or polyunsaturated fats. If your child remains on the diet, you should expect to visit the clinic on a yearly or more frequent basis as needed.

Coming Off the Diet

Generally, your doctor will begin to discuss having your child come off the diet after using it for 2 years. However, if there has been vast, yet not complete control of seizures, you should know that families often elect to continue to use the diet, especially if they believe that their child has adapted well to it and is healthy. Some patients may remain on the diet for many years, but they need thoughtful follow-up with respect to nutrition and particularly bone health. Most families approach the diet as they would any other medical therapy, such as anticonvulsants. If you know the diet is working better than all the other medicines did, you don't want to have it changed.

Side Effects of the Diet

Many types of side effects (*adverse events*) have been seen in association with the diet, but these should not make you afraid to use the diet. These adverse side effects include *cardiomyopathy* (a heart disorder), *pancreatitis*, vitamin and mineral deficiencies, *Fanconi's anemia*, *reflux*, bruising, and perhaps increased infection. You need to make your child's physician aware of your child's illnesses, and you particularly need to communicate any sense that there has been a real decline in health. Physicians must be aware of these issues and should follow keto children closely, recognizing that their nutritional status is somewhat fragile.

Evidence is suggesting that your child might not grow well while she is on the diet, although most children experience "catch-up" growth once they are off the diet. This may be particularly important if your child is very young. The "borderline" adequate nutrition provided by the ketogenic diet is of particular concern as it affects bone health. Although you will be giving your child vitamins, minerals, and calcium supplements, calcium is often not well absorbed in the presence of diets that are very high in fats. Children on the keto diet might need other interventions to keep their bones strong, but scientists don't know what they are yet. Broken bones do occur more frequently in children on the diet, and physicians must be aware of this possibility, especially in very young children who appear fussy or in pain.

Variations of the Ketogenic Diet

The classic ketogenic diet, as envisioned by Wilder, has always been open to modification. This was true even during the first decade of its use, when Peterman, also at the Mayo Clinic, made the first changes to the original plan. Because no one is sure exactly why the ketogenic diet works, it is reasonable to assume that thoughtful clinicians will continue to make changes, tweaking one element or another to make it more successful, more palatable, or easier to use.

However, you should *never change the diet you have agreed to give* without consulting your doctor and dietician. They must be able to help you sort out whether there are dangers in the changes you want to make, and they must know what is being given so that they can help you thoughtfully determine what is helping or hurting your child. If they don't know what your child is eating, they will not know what may be contributing to either an effective or ineffective treatment.

One of the first major changes to the original ketogenic diet was the substitution of MCTs for the saturated fats like butter and cream. MCT fats do not contain the carbohydrates or proteins that are found in dairy products, so they allow somewhat greater variability in the diet—children can eat a wider variety of foods and make up the necessary fats by eating MCTs. However, the MCTs often make children feel bloated, and sometimes MCTs cause diarrhea. Substituting MCTs for dairy fats may not be as effective as the more classical approach using butter and cream, and MCT oil is also rather expensive. But, if your child has constipation, some MCT oil may be helpful.

Another variation to the original ketogenic diet was to minimize the length of the fast leading into the diet. Originally, children were fasted until they lost 10% of their body weight. This was gradually decreased, without any apparent loss in efficacy of the diet; currently, many centers use a 24- to 48-hour fast, while many other centers do not fast children at all. This may be very important to the acceptance of the diet by cultures that would see fasting as particularly cruel to children. The use of fasting remains controversial, but likely has some role in controlling seizures for some children.

Some studies have suggested that certain lipids, particularly *polyunsaturated fatty acids* (PUFAs) such as *docosahexaenoic acid* (DHA), should be increased in the ketogenic diet, since they play important roles in membrane formation, especially in the developing brain. Your dietician may want to help you add more of these to your child's foods.

Traditionally, the ketogenic diet is prescribed at a 3:1 or 4:1 ratio in most Western countries, and some evidence suggests that these ratios are needed to achieve ketosis in these populations. However, as the diet is being adapted for use throughout the world, it must be sensitive to the cuisines of various cultures. Interestingly, it appears that somewhat lower ratios may be very effective in countries such as India, Thailand, and Korea, where rice is a critical staple of the diet. This is thought-provoking because it suggests many avenues of exploration, including an examination of whether the traditional adherence to the diet is necessary; whether certain food combinations, common in other countries, may be particularly helpful to seizure control; and whether genetic or race differences may affect the use of the diet.

Two other modifications are also being studied in the United States and may be important to a more widespread use of the diet. One modification involves blood glucose (sugar) levels. Some physicians believe that the keto diet is effective because it stabilizes blood glucose. On a normal diet, blood glucose can vary a great deal. A diet that is less strictly ketogenic, but uses foods with a low *glycemic index*, can offer a wider variety of foods. A better selection of foods may be more palatable and healthier over a longer period of use.

The other modification involves a variation of the Atkins diet, in which carbohydrates (carbs) are strictly limited while fat and proteins are not limited. This allows a much wider choice of foods and does not require foods to be carefully weighed and measured. Early studies suggest that the modified Atkins diet is quite effective, and it may also be a format that would be more acceptable to adults. You should inquire whether aspects of these less restrictive diets might be appropriate for your child.

The Future of the Ketogenic Diet

The medical community has become increasingly interested in implementing the ketogenic diet for seizure control, and in finding better ways to do it. In the last decade, many centers in the United States and around the world have developed ways to make the keto diet available to their patients, but many patients still have no access to it. Wider availability and easier methods will be important, as will the studies that demonstrate which patients are most likely to be helped. It will be important to know when the diet should be used earlier, rather than later, in treatment. Doctors must know that if your child has a particular type of seizure disorder, they should provide the keto diet immediately. And they also must know the reverse—that if your child has certain other types of seizure disorders, the diet would be a waste of time or even harmful. Scientists must continue to explore how the diet works, so that physicians can prescribe the diet to the right patients. It's important that those elements of the diet that make it effective are identified and used, and the potentially restrictive elements are abandoned. Some aspects of the diet may be important to certain types of epilepsy, while others may be important in different syndromes.

Many clues about epilepsy and its treatment are waiting to be uncovered. Until then, there are situations when you should consider using the ketogenic diet or one of its variations:

▶ When seizures are not controlled after trials of two appropriate medications.

▶ When seizures are controlled, but excessive side effects occur.

▶ If your child has one of the catastrophic childhood epilepsies (tuberous sclerosis, infantile spasms).

STEROIDS, NUTRITION, AND ALTERNATIVE THERAPIES

Steroids

The term *steroids* is used in medicine to describe a variety of different hormones that have similar chemical structures. These compounds serve a number of important functions. One group of these hormones are called the *corticosteroids* because they are produced by the *adrenal cortex* (glands above the kidneys). A subgroup of these corticosteroids are called *glucocorticoids* because they can influence how the body handles glucose (or sugar) metabolism. Glucocorticoids also have potent *anti-inflammatory* effects, and some can act directly on the brain. Two medicines in this class that are used for treatment of childhood epilepsies are *prednisone* and *prednisolone*. Both can potentially reduce seizures in younger children and are used to treat hard-to-control seizures that have failed treatment with other conventional drugs. Since these compounds are steroids, they can have other actions on the body that may be unfavorable. These include, but are not limited to, an increased risk of stomach ulcers, increased blood sugar levels, a predisposition to infections, and the development of high blood pressure. All these side effects can be treated, particularly if detected early, so judicious monitoring during administration of the drugs is very important. Monitoring includes general physical screening examinations that include a measurement of *vital signs* (weight, height, temperature, pulse, respiratory rate, and blood pressure), urinary dipsticks for glucose monitoring, and periodic examination of the stool for *occult* (hidden) blood.

Adrenocorticotrophic hormone (ACTH), another treatment in this class of drugs, is a very potent stimulator of adrenal function. This compound increases the body's own natural glucocorticoid production and has been the treatment of first choice for infantile spasms in the United States for the past half-century. A recent study just completed in England showed that ACTH is slightly more useful when compared to another more modern treatment (namely, vigabatrin) in cases of infantile spasms of unknown cause. In most cases, ACTH and vigabatrin were equivalent, particularly when long-term outcome was considered. The side-effects of ACTH are the same as those of any steroids, but older studies performed on ACTH showed some very serious side effects and even deaths occurred with the prolonged use of high doses of ACTH. For this reason, ACTH treatment must be closely monitored at all times. In addition, infants on ACTH should have careful screening for *heart disease* and should avoid contact with persons with infectious illnesses because the use of ACTH may suppress the immune system and reduce the body's ability to fight disease.

Nutrition

The ketogenic diet can be very effective in its ability to control or reduce seizures in some patients. Epilepsy patients often ask if other dietary changes, other than the strict ketogenic diet, can be beneficial. To date, no evidence suggests that simple alterations in diet, without producing ketosis, are beneficial for controlling seizures. In animal models, calorie restriction is helpful, but this is not practical for most people, and is particularly not relevant in children, in whom it is critical to ensure that enough dietary fuel is provided for normal daily activities and growth.

A balanced diet and a multivitamin are two of those undeniably good things, like mother and apple pie, that are widely recommended for everyone. Our dietician has the following advice: Everyone should eat three meals per day, with one or two snacks throughout the day. Starting every day with a well-balanced breakfast will help to fuel the body first thing in the morning. Every meal should include a good balance of whole grains, fruits, vegetables, and low-fat dairy products. Eating a variety of foods is a key component for good nutrition. Intentionally make every food on your plate a different color to increase the amount of nutrients consumed. In general, foods with bright and deep colors (reds, yellows, greens) contain a plethora of vitamins and minerals essential to a healthy diet. It is always better to try to get the vitamins that the body needs by eating the proper foods; however, when taking certain medications, it might be necessary to supplement the diet with specific nutrients.

Individuals taking anticonvulsant medications have some added special dietary considerations. Publications dating back to the 1970s raised concerns of *osteomalacia* or bone weakness caused by the use of anticonvulsant medications. The risks are higher in postmenopausal women, those who are institutionalized, or in individuals who are not walking. Routine evaluation and supplementation with extra vitamin D and calcium has been recommended by many neurologists, but there is as yet no widespread agreement on the optimal approach. *Folate* supplementation is particularly important for women of childbearing potential, as maternal folate levels may be depleted by medication and folate is important to protect against birth defects, including neural tube abnormalities.

Certain children have *pyridoxine-responsive seizures*, that are improved by treatment with vitamin B_6. Given the benign nature of a brief trial of B_6 and the remarkable impact on seizure control in some children, this should always be considered when refractory seizures are present. Vitamin E (400 IU per day) has been endorsed by some, but *blinded studies* failed to show a clear benefit. In the neonatal nursery, supplementation with B$_6$, pyridoxal phosphate, and folinic acid should be tried in all cases of refractory seizures.

Research has shown that diets high in polyunsaturated fats (typical of Mediterranean cuisine) are beneficial in certain neurologic diseases, particularly those in which chronic inflammation plays some role. To the extent that inflammation may be present in certain forms of epilepsy, diets high in polyunsaturated fats might be expected to be of some marginal benefit, but this has yet to be studied.

Relaxation and Alternative Stress Relievers

People with epilepsy report numerous triggers for their seizures, some of which appear to be highly individualized. Some common seizure triggers include poor sleep hygiene, fevers or illness, flashing lights (photosensitivity), and certain foods. The association between stress and seizures is not clearly documented, yet patients have often reported an increase in seizures when stressed. Stress can manifest in many different ways, including altering sleep patterns, decreasing or increasing appetite, and increasing the risk of infection. Therefore, a person with epilepsy who is stressed may experience a lower *seizure threshold* than another person with epilepsy who is practicing some basic stress-management strategies. Our epilepsy center social worker, Sarah Ahlm has the following recommendations:

> Some stress management strategies include exercising regularly and maintaining healthy eating habits. Exercise regimens can be fairly individualized, but can include cardio training, yoga, and walking. It is important to be aware of seizures precautions and the side effects of medications when choosing an exercise program. For example, if someone is experiencing decreased sweating due to an antiepileptic medication, vigorous cardio workouts would not be encouraged because of the risk of overheating. Likewise, a person with epilepsy should not swim laps alone or participate in competitive boxing tournaments.

Epilepsy can often cause people to feel a loss of control and therefore increased anxiety and depression. *Biofeedback* or *neurofeedback* involves the use of some instrument (like an electroencephalogram [EEG] that measures brain rhythms) to provide feedback. In one scenario, a practitioner evaluates a patient's EEG and then employs relaxation techniques, music, and/or computer games to help the patient to modulate his brain rhythms. Biofeedback can be useful in reducing stress and sometimes in reducing seizures. However, biofeedback can be time-consuming as well as expensive and therefore its use should be evaluated on an individual basis.

Other self-care strategies that can help with stress management include support groups, counseling, and recreational activities. When evaluating an appropriate stress-management program, it is important to look at your needs as they relate to the stress in your life. If you are feeling isolated by your seizures, and this is causing you to feel depressed, support groups or counseling might be an appropriate stress-management strategy. A person who is feeling isolated might also enjoy joining a bowling league or an art class to meet other people and integrate into the community. Having a psychological evaluation and treatment can help people get to the root of anxiety and depression, which may improve the *quality of life* as well as seizure control for an individual with epilepsy.

People with seizures report a decreased quality of life when compared with their peers. Actively employing stress-management strategies may help improve quality of life and seizure control. Remember, the key to managing stress is individualizing a program and following through with that self-care plan.

Other Alternatives Therapies

Complementary and Alternative Therapies in Epilepsy

Over the past decade, more and more patients and families have been using complementary and alternative medications to improve their health and to treat epilepsy. It is estimated that almost 50% of patients with chronic diseases use alternative treatments. In the United States, about 20% of people taking prescription medications also take herbal remedies or high-dose vitamins. There is a natural tendency to trust herbs because they are "natural" and, therefore "safer" than traditionally pharmaceutical drugs. However, it's important to realize that just because a treatment is "natural" does not mean it is "better" or "safer." The benefits—and risks—of any of these therapies is unknown, because few scientific studies have looked at their safety and how well these treatments work.

More important than the potential benefits of natural products, these forms of treatment may carry certain risks. These risks include the possible direct toxic effects of the preparations and their ingredients. Another risk is that, since these substances are not regulated by the U.S. *Food and Drug Administration* (FDA), toxic impurities, such as herbicides, may be present. Finally, herbs can interfere with the way other medicines, including anticonvulsant drugs, work. Your doctor must be aware of any herbs, supplements, or other alternative treatments that you are taking, to prevent dangerous interactions between your antiepileptic (or other prescription) medications and the alternative treatment.

Very few studies have addressed the use of herbs for the treatment of epilepsy, and most of those studies have involved animals. Over 100 compounds from around the world have been tested, but only a small number of human studies have been undertaken. The results are of questionable validity, however, because the studies involve small numbers of patients. Furthermore, they have not been done according to acceptable *scientific methods* and thus are not considered valid.

Many doctors believe that alternative therapies are acceptable as long as patients also continue taking traditional therapies, and the intended alternative and traditional therapies do not conflict. The problem is that we know very little about some of these unproven therapies and thus, the risk may outweigh the benefits. The most common forms of alternative therapies include herbs, vitamins, homeopathy, oils, and Chinese medicine. The information on the most common alternative therapies in the next sections has been partly obtained from the book *Complementary and Alternative Therapies for Epilepsy*, by Devinsky et al.

Herbs

Many herbs have been used to treat epilepsy. However, guidelines for these recommendations, studies to support their use, and which herbs are most commonly used to treat seizures are extremely difficult to find. The herbs detailed in the following paragraphs have been described as effective, or possibly effective, for the treatment of seizures.

The most popular selling herbs in the United States are ginkgo, St. John's wort, ginseng, garlic, echinacea, saw palmetto, kava, pycnogenol, cranberry, valerian root, evening primrose, bilberry, and milk thistle. Herbs used specifically for epilepsy are listed in Table 6.1.

TABLE 6.1
Herbs Used for Epilepsy

Valerian root	Chrysanthemum	European peony
Black cohosh	Burning bush	Ginger
Hyssop	Yew	Forskolin
Geranium	Scullcap	Calotropis
Passion flower	Kava	Lily-of-the-valley
Mugwort	Kelp	European mistletoe
Betony	Carline thistle	Tree of heaven
Flax seed oil	Lady's slipper	

Valerian Root

Valerian (*Valeriana officinalis*) is a herb native to Europe and Asia; it has been known as a sedative for thousands of years. It was probably named after the Roman emperor Valerian, who reigned from 253 to 260 A.D. It is an extremely popular herb in Western Europe, particularly in Germany and Russia. Research has shown it to improve the quality of sleep, and it is used for nervousness and insomnia. Although valerian is the most common herb prescribed for epilepsy, no significant animal or human proof of its usefulness exists for this disorder. Importantly, sudden discontinuation of valerian after chronic use can cause withdrawal symptoms such as confusion, similar to withdrawal from benzodiazepines or alcohol.

Kava

Kava (*Piper methysticum*) is widely used as a calming and sedative herb. Other names for Kava include *ava*, *awa*, *kava-kava*, *kawa*, *kew sakau*, *tonga*, and *yagona*.

Kava seems to have a positive effect on anxiety. Kava also appears to help with pain, muscle relaxation, and seizures, although these effects have not been scientifically proven in humans. Claims are made for the treatment of many conditions using kava, including asthma, depression, lack of sleep, and muscle spasms, pain. Kava should be avoided by pregnant and lactating women, children, and patients with kidney disease and blood disorders. This herb should not be used by depressed patients because the danger of suicide may be increased.

Kava can cause side effects such as sleepiness, loss of balance, headaches, dizziness, vision changes, diarrhea, and other problems. During the past several years, liver disease has also been reported.

American Hellebore

American hellebore (*Veratrum viride*) has been used to induce vomiting and for the treatment of headaches, pneumonia, and seizures. American hellebore is also known as *false hellebore*, *green hellebore*, *Indian poke*, and *itchweed*. This herb is a native to North America. American hellebore has multiple actions and can generally lower blood pressure, heart rate, and possibly respiratory rate in normal doses. However, this is a highly toxic compound and should be used with extreme caution.

Side effects include numbness of the extremities, paralysis of eye muscles, weakness, and seizures. Other side effects include nausea and vomiting, shortness of breath, increased salivation, and blood pressure problems. The plant is associated with serious potential for birth malformations, and thus it should not be used during pregnancy.

Blue Cohosh

Blue cohosh (*Caulophyllum thalictroides*) has been used as an anticonvulsant, and is also used to increase menstrual flow and induce labor. In the United States, nurse-midwives commonly use it in labor. The active agent, methylcytosine, is similar to but less potent than nicotine.

Synonyms for blue cohosh are blue ginseng, caulophyllum, papoose toot, squawroot, and yellow ginseng. The herb can cause diarrhea, stomach cramps, and chest pain.

Mistletoe

Mistletoe (*Viscum album*; *Phoradendron serotinum*) is also known as *all-heal*, *birdlime*, *devil's fuge*, *European mistletoe*, *golden bough*, and *viscum*. Mistletoe is widely used, despite its known toxic effects. It is used as remedy for various ailments; however, this is a highly toxic substance. Mistletoe can cause cardiac, brain, and gastrointestinal problems.

Although one study in animals showed some protective effect against seizure-causing agents, no clinical studies have been done on its use as an antiepileptic drug. Mistletoe can cause sedation, seizures, heart problems, low blood pressure, and liver damage, among other side effects.

Scullcap

Scullcap (*Scutellaria lateriflora*), also known as *helmet flower* and *hoodwort*, is a North American herb used as a nerve tonic for the treatment of restlessness, poor sleep, spasms, and alcohol addiction. It has been used to treat epilepsy, but no scientific studies and experiments support its use. Scullcap may be used as the dried herb or liquid extract. Side effects may include giddiness, confusion, and twitching. Preparations of scullcap may be contaminated with other herbs, which may cause liver damage. It should be used with great caution during pregnancy and lactation.

Marijuana

Marijuana (*Cannabis sativa*) has wide illegal use in the general population. The herb has several potential medicinal properties, including antiepileptic effects and as a medication to relieve nausea. Marijuana has variable effects, being antiseizure in some animal models and human forms of epilepsy (partial epilepsy), but with evidence that it can provoke seizures in generalized epilepsies. Several small human studies in epilepsy found an insignificant reduction in seizures; however, the study populations were small, and low doses of cannabidiol (CBD; one of the active ingredients in marijuana) were used.

As with alcohol, seizures may occur upon sudden discontinuation after regular use. The bottom line on marijuana and epilepsy remains problematic, and no general statements can be made about how useful it is to treat epilepsy. In addition, marijuana use is presently illegal, and its long-term use is associated with other health problems, such as breathing, nervous system, and hormonal disorders.

Chinese Medicine

The medical therapies of China, Japan, and Asia are based on herbs or mixtures of herbs rather than on single agents. Although used for thousand of years, little evidence from scientific studies shows that these herbal mixtures are useful for the treatment of epilepsy. There are few comparative studies using traditional Chinese herbs.

Qingyangsen, a mixture of Chinese roots, showed improvement in 30% of patients, without causing side effects. In another study, the herbal preparation *Zhenxianling*, which contains peach flower buds, human placenta, and other ingredients, showed a more than 75% reduction in seizures in 66% of patients. Two Asian herbal mixtures of the same nine herbs have been studied in the treatment of seizures: Japanese *shosaikoto* (or *saiko-keishi-to*) and Chinese *chai-hu-keui-chi-tang* (a *bupleurum-cinnamon* combination). In one study, saiko-keishi-to resulted in seizure control in 25% of patients for at least 10 months. However, shosaikoto has also been associated with the development of allergic lung inflammation and death, as well as liver injury; these are rare side effects with shosaikoto, but they cast doubt on its general safety.

Essentials Oils

Essential oils are highly concentrated extracts from a variety of plants used for aromatherapy, massage, and other purposes. Essential oils contain many chemicals, and these chemicals can gain entry into the body and the brain through the skin or the lungs.

Several essential oils have been reported to cause seizures either in patients who never had a seizure before or to make seizures worse in patients with epilepsy. The essential oils of greatest concern are eucalyptus, fennel, hyssop, pennyroyal rosemary, sage, savin, turpentine, and wormwood. Wormwood is the active ingredient in the alcoholic beverage absinthe, which contains the convulsant chemical thujone. These essential oils should be avoided by people who have seizures.

Melatonin

Although melatonin is not an herb, its use and popularity deserves mention. Melatonin is normally produced by the pineal gland, which is located in the middle of the brain, and it is secreted to the base of the brain where it likely promotes sleep. Removing the pineal gland in animals may produce seizures. A small number of children with light-sensitive epilepsy have low melatonin levels. Melatonin is marketed as a dietary supplement because it is found in some plants. It is not FDA-approved or regulated.

Melatonin has some reported anticonvulsant effects, but it has been shown to both increase *and* decrease seizure frequency. Most reports suggest that it may be more effective in children. Melatonin may improve sleep quality, and because sleep has such an important effect on seizures, the improvement in sleep quality alone may reduce seizures. Doses in the range of 2 to 5 mg are commonly used, but no scientific evidence support this use. Concerns exist regarding its adverse effects. These include drowsiness, sleep disruption, nightmares, low sperm count, and abdominal pain. Concerns also exist regarding effects on puberty, because animals given melatonin have delayed sexual maturation. Melatonin may also cause *vasoconstriction*, a particular concern for patients with coronary artery disease.

Seizures Provoked by Herbs

Although herbal medicines are used to treat seizures, several herbal medicines may actually worsen or provoke seizures. Many of these herbs have compounds that are stimulants and thus can increase the likelihood of seizures. The following herbs should be avoided or, if taken, you should tell your doctor about them.

Ephedra

Ephedra is a traditional medicine that has been used for many years in Asia and by Native Americans in the Midwest. The main active ingredient in ephedra is *ephedrine*. Ephedrine is a stimulant, and some reports have surfaced of people experiencing seizures after taking ephedra. Ephedra should be avoided by people who have experienced seizures.

Caffeine

Caffeine is one of the most commonly used stimulants. Coffee and tea have caffeine in them, but several other foods, beverages, and herbs also contain caffeine. Cocoa, which is the main ingredient in chocolate, contains caffeine, as does the cola nut, which is used to make soft drinks. Two other popular drinks containing large amounts of caffeine are maté and guarana. Maté is a bushy plant whose leaves are used to prepare a sort of tea that is very popular in Argentina, Paraguay, and Brazil. Guarana is made from the seed of a climbing shrub that grows in the Amazon. Guarana is popular in soft drinks beverages in South America.

Caffeine acts by stimulating the release of neurotransmitters in the brain, thus increasing brain activity and creating a mentally stimulating effect. Caffeine can prolong seizure activity in several animal studies. Caffeine can also prolong seizures in people who are given electroshock treatments for depression. So, it is probably best for people with seizures to avoid or at least minimize their use of caffeine-containing products.

Ginkgo

Ginkgo (*Ginkgo biloba*) is a popular herbal medicine used to improve memory. It is uncertain how ginkgo improves memory, but it may increase brain *acetylcholine* levels, an important brain chemical that begins to deteriorate as aging occurs.

The FDA has received reports of people experiencing seizures after taking ginkgo. However, it is difficult to determine whether ginkgo actually caused these seizures or whether this was due to chance. It may be safer for people diagnosed with epilepsy to avoid taking gingko until more is known about its effects.

Ginseng

Ginseng is a popular drink in Asia. Ginseng has a reputation for treating many different ailments, including memory loss. Although animal research indicates that ginseng may improve memory, very little research has been done to prove or disprove this in humans.

Ginseng activates the stress hormone system. Stress hormones can worsen seizures, and it may be best for people with epilepsy to avoid ginseng.

Evening Primrose and Borage

Evening primrose (*Oenothera biennis*) is used as an herbal remedy for premenstrual syndrome, although it is uncertain if it has any benefits. Borage (*Borago officinalis*) has a reputation for treating depression, inflammation, fevers, and coughs, but these effects have never been tested. Some research suggests that these herbs may reduce seizures; some suggest that they may increase them. It may be safest for people with seizures to avoid either.

RESOURCES FOR COMPLEMENTARY AND ALTERNATIVE MEDICINES

National Center for Complementary and Alternative Medicine
http:// nccam.nih.gov

Office of Dietary Supplement
http://odp.od.nih.gov/ods

Centre for Complementary Health Studies
Exeter University, Exeter EX4 4RG
www.exeter.ac.uk

PhytoNet Home Page
www.escop.com

FREQUENTLY ASKED QUESTIONS

Q How soon will I know if the ketogenic diet is going to work?

A It seems to vary a great deal. There are some children for whom it is clear that the diet will work almost immediately. Seizures seem to evaporate as they are fasted, and virtually disappear before they are discharged from the hospital. This certainly doesn't happen as often as we would wish, and parents shouldn't be disappointed if they see other children initially doing better than their child. Parents are encouraged to work with the diet for about 3 months before they abandon it. Rarely, children improve even more gradually, and the full effect of the diet isn't seen for as long as 6 months. Generally, encouraging signs along the way enable families and children to persist. These include changes such as shorter seizures or the child having more energy and being more alert. During that time, many adjustments can be made that make all the difference: Calories are increased or decreased depending on the nutritional needs of the child; the ratio can be changed to try to induce better ketosis; or better control may even involve decreasing anticonvulsant medications. A variety of strategies may maximize the effect of the diet, which is why it is important to work closely with experienced dieticians and physicians.

Q If my child starts the keto diet, can his anticonvulsants be discontinued right away?

A Many families choose the ketogenic diet because they see it as a more natural way to control seizures. They are frightened about the side effects of medications and, in many instances, they believe that these side effects are badly effecting their child's behavior or learning ability. These parents believe that, if only the medications were stopped, their children would function more normally. However, the ketogenic diet is certainly not a "natural" way of eating, and side effects certainly are associated with its use. Generally, it is not wise to stop anticonvulsants as soon as the diet is initiated. Some medications, like phenobarbital, probably should be reduced. Others, like topiramate and zonisamide, are associated with an increased risk of kidney stones and, although no evidence suggests that children on these medications and the ketogenic diet have an even higher risk of stones, these medications are routinely tapered first. Studies have shown that children can be tapered off (or *weaned*) from some of their medication even during the first month of the diet, but parents are typically encouraged to keep medications steady until the diet has been stabilized. That means that most medications aren't tapered until the child has been on the diet for at least 1 to 3 months. There are many advantages to weaning a child off anticonvulsants that have not been successful, including ending or avoiding unpleasant side effects and saving money. You should develop a plan with your treatment team that is committed to trying to eliminate medications that are not clearly helpful to your child.

Q Is my child really getting enough to eat on the keto diet? She seems to be hungry, but she doesn't always finish the meals that I make for her.

A Many issues are involved in this question. Children won't voluntarily starve themselves. If your child is not eating, first make certain that you've worked with your child's dietician to find meal plans that are satisfying and appropriate for your child. If the meal plans are appropriate, but behavioral issues continue, such as fights over mealtime, then you might also need the help of a behavioral therapist. Sometimes, just substituting another family member to supervise meal time helps by removing the upsetting interactions between parent and child.

If your child seems genuinely hungry all the time, her dietician can sometimes add more bulk to the meal so that your child will feel fuller. This also involves making sure your child is consuming all the liquids she needs as well.

The most important issue in this question, however, is whether your child is getting adequate nutrition. This is best answered by knowing whether your child is healthy and has enough energy to participate in all her various activities. If your child is not getting ill, is growing at a slowed but steady pace, and can do the things expected of her in school and at play, then she is likely getting enough to eat. (It may not look like enough to eat on a big plate, but it may look much better on a special, smaller plate reserved only for the child on the diet.)

Parents must maintain a positive attitude that the nutrition they are providing is really right for the child. Too many children are overfed. Love doesn't depend on the size of a meal.

Q Does stress cause children to have seizures?

A We are often asked this question by parents, perhaps for a variety of different reasons. It may be that some parents harbor feelings of guilt or concern that something they did brought on seizures. In other circumstances, it may be that parents are concerned that they are "pushing the child too hard," either in school or with regard to other expectations. Finally, other family strife may also be present.

All these concerns are important to address. It is not possible, to the best of our knowledge, to directly cause seizures in the vast majority of cases. There are very rare seizures that occur in response to specific environmental stimuli (*reflex seizures*) but, by and large, parents cannot cause seizures by their actions.

A natural reaction on behalf of most parents is to become overprotective and somewhat overindulgent once their child has shown a vulnerability to seizures. In this regard, it is helpful to keep in mind that children with epilepsy should be treated similarly to any other child, to the greatest extent possible. Appropriate discipline is actually helpful in providing the child with easily understood guidelines of acceptable behavior. Children like to know the limits and are reassured by understanding the rules. Overindulgence, for fear of creating a stressful situation, becomes counterproductive in the long run. If this overindulgence leads to bad behavior, your child may have problems socializing with others or doing well in school. In the long run, this issue ends up producing more stress for the child.

Family problems, like unhappy marriages or other dysfunctional relationships, are important to recognize. Although these are obviously not the direct cause of seizures, they may contribute to misunderstanding and often seem to create the very opposite of a therapeutic environment. Family counseling may be appropriate and beneficial in these cases.

School-related problems can cause substantial stress, both for the child and her family. Fortunately, many resources can be brought to bear on the situation. A useful tip is to schedule time with the child's educators to express concern and to learn more about the school's assessment. If significant concerns are present, a formal evaluation can be called for, including *neuropsychological testing*. Sometimes, all that is required are some adaptations. In other circumstances, more resources are needed, even a change in the school setting. *Individualized education plans* (IEPs) summarize the results of the evaluation and make specific recommendations. These evaluations are commonly repeated every 3 years, but can be updated more frequently, if the need arises. Educators benefit from detailed medical information that is specific to the child. An up-to-date medical summary is very helpful information to have at the IEP. An alignment between the abilities of the child and her scholastic expectations can lead to reduction in stress and improvement in the child's self-esteem.

Q What vitamins or other supplements should I take if I am taking antiepileptic drugs?

A Talk to your doctor. In general, a multivitamin is appropriate. Folate is particularly important for women of child-bearing age. Vitamin D and calcium may also be indicated, particularly in those at risk for bone problems.

As a special note of caution, herbal supplements may have potent effects, particularly on drug metabolism. It is important to inform your doctor and pharmacist of concurrent supplements so that they can check for possible drug-on-drug interactions.

My Notes

_____

_____

_____

_____

_____

7

SEIZURES AND EPILEPSY IN CHILDREN

Recognition, Diagnosis, and Treatment

Key Points

▶ Because of the immature condition of the baby's brain, neonatal seizures often appear different from seizures in older individuals.

▶ Febrile seizures are seizures that occur in association *only* with fever, in children between the ages of 18 months and 3 years, and without evidence of a serious infection (such as meningitis) or other central nervous system cause.

▶ *Benign rolandic epilepsy* (BRE) is the most common type of childhood epilepsy in children between ages 2 and 12 years. Affected children experience seizures soon after falling asleep, during daytime naps, or upon awakening.

▶ Children are especially vulnerable to the side effects of certain medications and, conversely, seem resistant to others.

NEONATAL SEIZURES

SEIZURES ARE MORE COMMON in newborn infants (*neonates*) than in older children or adults. Seizures occur in 1 to 5 babies per 1,000. The incidence is highest in very-low-birth-weight infants (those who weigh less than 1,500 grams or about 3 pounds).

Newborns are more likely to have seizures for several reasons, including an immature nervous system, birth defects affecting the brain, biochemical or *metabolic problems*, and many diseases that affect newborn infants. Although most brain development occurs before birth, further developmental changes happen during early childhood, leaving the newborn especially susceptible to seizures. These changes include *myelination* (insulation) of nerve fibers, formation of new connections (*synapses*) between neurons, and the normal loss of some neurons (*apoptosis*), as well as changes in the balance between the chemicals called *neurotransmitters* that help to control the brain's activity.

Risk factors for neonatal seizures include:

▶ Premature age, especially infants born before 30 weeks of gestation
▶ Male gender
▶ *Intraventricular hemorrhage* (bleeding inside the ventricles of the brain)
▶ *Necrotizing enterocolitis*, a condition that causes parts of the infant's bowel to die, leading to infection (*sepsis*)
▶ *Patent ductus arteriosus*, a congenital heart defect that can affect brain circulation
▶ Lack of oxygen at birth and birth defects (mostly in full-term infants)

Types of Neonatal Seizures

Because of the immature condition of the baby's brain, neonatal seizures often appear different from seizures in older individuals. Neonatal seizures may be difficult to recognize, even by trained doctors and nurses. Without continuous *video-electroencephalogram* (video-EEG) monitoring, neonatal seizures may be misinterpreted as normal newborn behavior or missed altogether, especially if they lack outward signs. Unlike older individuals, newborns do not have typical, generalized tonic–clonic (grand mal) seizures.

Seizures in newborns can be classified into several types:

▶ *Clonic seizures* that are either *focal*, with repetitive jerking of a single region of the body (face, arm, trunk, or leg) or *multifocal*, involving several body regions.
▶ *Tonic seizures*, characterized by sustained stiffening of a limb or the whole body, lasting a few seconds.
▶ *Myoclonic seizures*, characterized by rapid jerks occurring singly or repeatedly.
▶ *Subtle seizures*, such as lip smacking or chewing; roving eye movements; eyes turned up, down, or to the side for a prolonged period (known as *eye deviation*); or eye opening and

staring. Infants may also manifest "bicycling" movements of the legs, "swimming" movements of the arms, or abrupt changes in pupil size or heart rate. Difficulty breathing (*apnea*) as the only sign of a seizure is uncommon and usually is caused by something else, such as a still-developing breath-regulation system, infection, or respiratory, cardiac, or metabolic disturbances. In near-term infants, apnea may be accompanied by other seizure phenomena such as eye deviation, eye opening, or repetitive mouth movements.

▶ *Subclinical seizures*, which are detected only by EEG, because they have no outward signs.

Diagnosis

Neonatal seizures are usually diagnosed when a caregiver identifies an unusual pattern of behavior, such as those just described. The most commonly used diagnostic procedure is the EEG, which records brain electrical activity and can determine whether the pattern is normal or abnormal. In the newborn, the EEG is typically recorded for at least an hour. However, this interval may be insufficient, and more prolonged video-EEG recording for hours or days may be required to make a positive diagnosis. Subtle seizures and certain seizure types may not have abnormalities detectable in the scalp-recorded EEG. In this situation, the trained eye of a neurologist may be necessary to recognize if seizures are occurring or not. In contrast, sick newborns, many of whom are paralyzed and on breathing machines, may have seizures that can only be detected by EEG.

Additional tests to determine the cause of the seizures include blood tests to check for abnormalities in sugar and *electrolyte* (sodium, calcium, magnesium) levels, which can be corrected relatively easily. Additional tests for metabolic disorders may be necessary in some newborns. Examples include blood tests for lactic and pyruvic acid levels; or blood or urine testing for amino acids and urine organic acids. A *lumbar puncture* (spinal tap) can check spinal fluid sugar and protein levels. A family history of seizures, especially during the newborn period or infancy, should be identified because genetic factors can be responsible for seizures in the newborn.

Imaging tests, such as *ultrasound, computed tomography* (CT), or *magnetic resonance imaging* (MRI) scans of the brain can show malformations or other structural abnormalities such as hemorrhage (bleeding in the brain), enlarged ventricles, birth defects, or stroke. Ultrasound of the head can be performed at the bedside, but CT and MRI scans require that the infant be transported by a medical team to the radiology department. MRI scans, which take a much longer time than CT scans, are usually done when the infant is medically stable.

Treatment

The treatment of neonatal seizures depends in part on establishing the cause. Biochemical disturbances are common in newborns with seizures, and some are easily corrected. Phenobarbital and fosphenytoin (Cerebyx) are primary agents administered intravenously for recurrent seizures. To stop seizures quickly, physicians may also administer lorazepam (Ativan) or diazepam (Valium) by vein, by mouth, or rectally. Less commonly used antiepileptic drugs (AEDs) include valproic acid (Depakene), lamotrigine (Lamictal), levetiracetam (Keppra), topiramate (Topamax), and zonisamide (Zonegran). Although no AED has been extensively tested in newborns, and none have been approved by the U.S. Food and Drug Administration (FDA) for use in infants, physicians use these medications because of their known safety and effectiveness in older children and adults.

Newborns with extremely frequent or prolonged seizures are referred to as having *status epilepticus*, a life-threatening condition that requires aggressive treatment with antiepileptic medications, usually in an intensive-care setting.

Outcome

Medical treatment with phenobarbital and phenytoin stops seizures in approximately 70% of children. Status epilepticus that does not respond to medications is particularly serious in the newborn and carries a high risk of death.

Fortunately, most infants with easily correctable metabolic disturbances or brain hemorrhage have a good outcome and do need antiepileptic medication. Prompt recognition and treatment of more serious metabolic disorders, like certain chemical imbalances or vitamin deficiencies (for example, vitamin B_6), can also result in normal outcome. Infants who have a few isolated seizures after experiencing a lack of oxygen (*hypoxic–ischemic injury*) or mild infection may have an excellent outcome, without the need for antiepileptic medication. Quite often, infants are discharged from the nursery without seizure medications, or their AEDs are stopped by 1 or 2 months of age, if there have been no further seizures.

Two-thirds of infants having frequent neonatal seizures or status epilepticus are at risk for serious problems, including cerebral palsy or developmental delay. In a large group of newborns followed from birth to 7 years, 61% developed epilepsy, most within the first 2 years of life. The outcome is poor in children with severe brain malformations and certain metabolic disorders.

FEBRILE SEIZURES

Febrile seizures are seizures that occur in association only with fever, in children between the ages of 18 months and 3 years, and without evidence of a serious infection (such as meningitis) or other central nervous system cause. This definition is important, because febrile seizures are not related to infections of the brain or nervous system and are not true epilepsy, and because affected children are *not* at risk for seizures unless they have a fever.

Febrile seizures run in families. They are approximately two to three times more common among the family members of affected children, and having an affected parent increases the risk of occurrence. (A higher incidence of epilepsy has been reported in close relatives, such as parents or brothers and sisters.) Ninety percent of children with febrile seizures will have them within the first 3 years of life, 4% before 6 months, and 6% after 3 years of age. Approximately half of these seizures appear during the second year of life, with a peak between 18 and 24 months.

A febrile seizure typically occurs early in the course of an infectious illness, usually on the rising phase of the temperature curve. Rectal temperatures often exceed 102°F (39.2°C), and one-fourth of seizures occur at temperatures above 104°F (40.2°C). However, febrile seizures aren't more likely to appear the higher the child's temperature, and they are usually uncommon in the later stages of a fever-producing illness.

Febrile seizures are typically associated with common childhood illnesses, usually viral upper respiratory, middle ear, and gastrointestinal infections. Bacterial infections, including pneumonia and meningitis, are less common causes.

Types of Febrile Seizures

Simple Febrile Convulsions

Simple febrile convulsions are single "events" lasting less than 15 minutes. These seizures don't involve any weakness of a limb, vision changes, or other serious effects. They usually involve shaking, jerking, or kicking movements, and the child may appear to lose consciousness briefly. These simple febrile convulsions occur in normal children who do not have brain-related conditions, defects, or injuries. Between 80% and 90% of all febrile seizures are simple episodes. Because most tests done on these children will come back with normal results, most doctors are very careful not to order too many unnecessary blood tests or brain scans. Hospitalization is rarely necessary.

Complex Febrile Seizures

The concept of a "complex" febrile seizure originated with studies indicating that some patient- and seizure-related variables are associated with higher rates of developing epilepsy at a later stage. These include seizures that last longer than 15 minutes, seizures with a focal pattern, seizures that recur within 24 hours, seizures occurring in a child who has a brain or nervous system abnormality, and seizures occurring in a child who has a parent or sibling with seizures that are not related to fevers (*afebrile seizures*).

In general, complex febrile seizures have a less favorable outcome than simple febrile convulsions. Seventeen percent of neurologically impaired children with complex febrile seizures develop epilepsy by the third decade of life, compared with 2.5% of children who lack risk factors. If a child has focal seizures, multiple episodes, and prolonged seizures, she has nearly a 50% chance of developing afebrile seizures later on.

Recurrence of Febrile Seizures

Approximately one-third of patients with a first febrile seizure will experience additional attacks, and one-half will have a third seizure. Only 9% experience three or more attacks.

Age at onset is the most important predictor of febrile seizure recurrence. One-half of all infants younger than 1 year of age at the time of their first febrile seizure will have a recurrence, compared with 20% of children older than 3 years of age. Young age at onset, febrile seizures in a first-degree relative, low-grade fever in the emergency department, and a brief interval between fever onset and seizure onset are all indicators of febrile seizure recurrence. Recurrences generally occur within 1 year but are no more likely in children who have had a complex than a simple febrile seizure.

Treatment

When your child has a fever, it's important to give her anti-fever medications, such as acetaminophen (Tylenol), and tepid sponge baths to control her temperature. Unfortunately, in some children, it's hard to tell when they have a fever until they have a seizure. It's important to watch for other signs of infection, such as lack of appetite, diarrhea, or rash and consult your doctor immediately.

Although medication can be given to *stop* a febrile seizure, AEDs should not be given to children to *prevent* simple febrile seizures. Recurrent febrile seizures and later afebrile epilepsy are both fortunately rare occurrences, and the risks of a child routinely taking an AED far outweigh the benefit in the case of febrile seizures.

The use of medication is sometimes considered for complex febrile seizures that carry an increased risk for later epilepsy. However, even seemingly life-threatening seizures must be treated cautiously. Since neurologic impairment and death are extremely unlikely, most children do not require long-term medication.

Febrile seizures often stop by the time a child is examined in the emergency room. If the seizure continues, the physician can give intravenous medication to stop the seizure. At home, rectally administered diazepam gel is safe and easy to use. Respiratory depression (shallow breathing) can occur, but this is rare.

COMMON CHILDHOOD EPILEPSY SYNDROMES

In a discussion of childhood epilepsy syndromes, it's important to understand the difference between *epileptic seizures*, *epilepsy*, and *epilepsy syndromes*.

Epileptic seizures are the symptoms resulting from an abnormal electrical discharge in the brain. There are many types of seizures, and children may have more than one seizure type.

Epilepsy is a disorder in which an individual has recurrent epileptic seizures.

Epilepsy syndrome refers to a cluster of specific signs and symptoms occurring in addition to epileptic seizures in the same child. For example, children with Lennox-Gastaut syndrome have multiple seizure types but are also mentally retarded and have a specific EEG pattern. In some, but not all syndromes, the specific cause, type of seizures, and outcome are well established. An example is *juvenile myoclonic epilepsy* (JME), which is known to be a genetic disease starting in adolescence or young adulthood, featuring specific seizure types that persist throughout the person's life. Other epilepsy syndromes may not have a clear cause, or may have several causes. The Lennox-Gastaut syndrome may occur after lack of oxygen at birth (*asphyxia*), from a head injury or metabolic disorder, or from many other factors.

Common Epilepsy Syndromes

Benign rolandic epilepsy (BRE) is the most common type of childhood epilepsy in children between ages 2 and 12 years. Affected children experience seizures soon after falling asleep, during daytime naps, or upon awakening. Focal motor seizures are most common, while generalized tonic–clonic seizures are rare. Seizures often involve the tongue, lips, and mouth and produce drooling and vocalizations. Younger children (under 5 years) are more likely to have a *hemiconvulsion* affecting one side of the body or a grand mal seizure. Their neurologic examination is normal.

The EEG helps confirm the diagnosis of BRE by demonstrating epileptic electrical activity in the central and temporal regions of the brain. This activity increases during sleep and has a characteristic appearance. Brain scans are typically normal, so that, when these EEG patterns are present, imaging studies are often unnecessary.

Children with BRE may experience a single seizure (50% will have fewer than five), or seizures may occur more regularly. BRE is believed to be a genetic disorder. However, although many children (and their siblings) show the characteristic EEG patterns, 90% never have seizures. BRE epileptiform discharges are common in children undergoing EEGs to evaluate other conditions. Unless they are having seizures, these EEG findings should be ignored.

Medical treatment may not be necessary when seizures are rare and occur during sleep. If treatment is indicated, BRE seizures are easily controlled with medications like gabapentin (Neurontin), carbamazepine (Tegretol or Carbatrol), or oxcarbazepine (Trileptal). In Europe, sulthiame (Ospolot) or valproic acid (Depakote) are also used. The outcome of BRE is excellent, as both seizures and EEG abnormalities disappear between ages 12 and 16 years. AEDs can be withdrawn if no seizures are observed for 2 years. Even if the EEG shows persistent epileptic activity, most neurologists will still attempt to wean the child from medication.

Childhood absence epilepsy is the second most common form of childhood epilepsy. It usually begins in healthy children between the ages of 4 to 10 years. It is genetically inherited. Absence seizures (often called petit mal seizures) consist of brief episodes of staring and arrest of ongoing activity lasting 3 to 10 seconds, but these episodes may occasionally last as long as 20 or 30 seconds. Absence seizures may be accompanied by lip-smacking, blinking, or gestural movements, and they typically occur many times daily. Shorter seizures may go unrecognized or be mistaken for inattentiveness, and school performance may suffer.

Seizures are usually noticed in the daytime and can be evoked by *hyperventilation* (rapid breathing). Grand mal seizures are rare, and are more commonly observed in older children. Absence seizures in children between 10 and 17 years represent a different disorder due to their more frequent association with grand mal (80%) and myoclonic (15%) seizures.

The EEG is almost always abnormal, even in children taking AEDs. Hyperventilation may be employed in the doctor's office or EEG laboratory to start an absence seizure and confirm the diagnosis. Consciousness is impaired during seizures that last longer than 3 seconds, but with even longer seizures, children may become partly responsive.

Unlike BRE, where treatment may not be required, absence seizures should be treated promptly because these seizures impair attention and learning and compromise overall safety on the playground, school, home, or street. The most commonly used medications include ethosuximide (Zarontin), valproic acid (Depakene or Depakote), and lamotrigine (Lamictal). Newer potential drugs include topiramate (Topamax) and zonisamide (Zonegran). Most absence seizures can be controlled. Hyperventilation testing and repeat EEG studies may be used to verify the effectiveness of treatment.

After a seizure-free interval of 2 years, medication may be safely discontinued. Most children outgrow absence seizures, but a small proportion continues to require medication and may evolve into juvenile myoclonic epilepsy.

Juvenile myoclonic epilepsy (JME) starts during adolescence, typically between 12 and 18 years of age. It is a genetic disorder. Myoclonic seizures predominate, consisting of abrupt jerks usually involving the shoulders and upper extremities. They typically occur in the morning after awakening. Myoclonic seizures may make the individual drop or fling objects from his hands. Grand mal seizures occur in over 90% of patients, and occur soon after waking in the morning. Repetitive myoclonic jerks can lead into a grand mal seizure. Jerking may be predominantly one-sided.

Patients with JME have normal neurologic examinations and normal brain MRI scans, but their EEGs reveals rapid *spike-wave discharges*. In approximately one-third of JME patients, seizures or EEG spike-wave discharges can be triggered by flickering lights. Absence seizures occur in 10% to 33% of patients with JME.

Effective seizure control is possible in over 90% of patients. Valproic acid (Depakote) is the most effective AED but is associated with weight gain and hormonal changes in women. Other medications such as topiramate (Topamax), zonisamide (Zonegran), lamotrigine (Lamictal), and levetiracetam (Keppra) are effective treatments and have fewer side effects. The treatment of JME is typically life-long, as attempts to reduce AEDs result in seizure recurrence in most individuals. It is important for patients to take their medications regularly, obtain adequate sleep, and refrain from using alcohol.

Infantile spasms (*West syndrome*) is an age-related epilepsy syndrome occurring in infants younger than 2 years. The peak incidence is between 3 and 7 years. There are many different causes, some of which occur prior to birth (brain malformations, infections while in the womb), at birth, or just after birth (lack of blood supply and oxygen, stroke, brain infections, trauma, brain tumors, metabolic and genetic disorders). *Tuberous sclerosis* is an additional cause. Brain scans are abnormal in about three-quarters of infants with West syndrome.

The spasms consist of an abrupt flexing of the arms, legs, and trunk, often followed by a more prolonged tonic phase lasting for about 2 seconds. Spasms typically occur numerous times over several minutes and "cluster" throughout the day, most often occurring while the child is falling asleep or waking up. Between spasms, infants appear quiet or irritable. Although 90% of children with infantile spasms are developmentally delayed prior to seizure onset, nearly all will show a loss of development once the spasms begin.

The EEG in West syndrome is very characteristic, showing multifocal spikes over both cerebral hemispheres and a disorganized high-voltage background—a pattern called *hypsarrhythmia*. Hypsarrhythmia typically evolves into other EEG patterns as the spasms transform into other seizure types. The majority of infants with West syndrome remain neurologically abnormal and continue to have seizures, but in 10% the spasms cease and the EEG returns to normal.

Prompt recognition and treatment of infantile spasms is mandatory. The most often recommended treatment is a course of ACTH hormone given by intramuscular injection, usually in addition to antiepileptic medications such as clonazepam (Klonopin), valproic acid (Depakene or Depakote), topiramate (Topamax), or zonisamide (Zonegran). Some infants respond to pyridoxine (vitamin B$_6$) or the *ketogenic diet*. Vigabatrin (Sabril) is a drug not yet approved in the United States that is also effective in controlling infantile spasms. Unfortunately, complete control of seizures is difficult to achieve, and less than 50% of infants are completely seizure-free. ACTH or other steroids such as prednisone may cause serious side effects.

Some infants with infantile spasms have a particular area of brain damage that causes their spasms, and surgical removal of the epileptic tissue may be the only way to stop the spasms.

Lennox-Gastaut syndrome (LGS) refers to the occurrence of multiple seizure types (most often generalized tonic, atonic, generalized tonic–clonic, myoclonic, or atypical absence seizures) in patients with mental retardation and a characteristic EEG consisting of slow spike-wave discharges. Seizures usually begin between ages 1 and 8 years. In contrast to the typical absence seizures seen in childhood absence epilepsy, the atypical absence seizures of LGS occur in neurologically and developmentally impaired children, often do not have an abrupt onset or end, and usually last longer than 15 seconds. LGS is produced by conditions similar to those associated with infantile spasms, but the cause is undetermined in nearly one-third of children. About 40% of LGS patients started out having infantile spasms. In addition to requiring an MRI and EEG, children with LGS should be evaluated for metabolic or *degenerative* illnesses of the brain. Seizures in LGS are often difficult to fully control with medications.

Temporal lobe epilepsy (TLE) in children differs from TLE in adults. Young children rarely describe *auras* occurring before their seizures start—such as abdominal sensations, nausea, altered taste, smell, déjà vu experiences, or visual or auditory hallucinations—but adult TLE patients often do. Children are more likely to have motor seizures, and infants and very young children are especially prone to spasms and myoclonic seizures—patterns that are rare in later life. Infants with temporal lobe seizures may also have a subtle reduction of activity (referred to as *hypomotor seizures*), pale skin, or changes in breathing.

In children younger than 6 years, malformations of the brain's *cerebral cortex*, including tumors, are common, while older children and adolescents usually have causes that are more similar to adults, such as *hippocampal sclerosis*. Hippocampal sclerosis is scarring of the temporal lobe, and it has been linked to prolonged febrile convulsions in infancy.

The EEG may show focal slowing and sharp waves in the temporal region in approximately half the cases, and the MRI is abnormal in nearly 80%. Treating with AEDs for partial seizures is effective in approximately half the children. TLE should be treated aggressively and, if seizures are not controlled in a reasonable time period, an evaluation for epilepsy surgery can be started. *Temporal lobectomy*, the removal of the diseased temporal lobe, leads to complete seizure freedom in 60% to 80% of children with TLE. If a temporal lobe tumor is present, early removal is advised because recurring seizures may lead to learning and behavioral problems.

Landau-Kleffner syndrome is characterized by the loss of previously acquired language and is frequently associated with behavioral and cognitive abnormalities. In the typical patient, a near-complete loss of spoken and understood language takes place slowly over a period of weeks or months between the ages of 18 months and 5 years. Affected children have autistic-like behavior, with a profound loss of attention. Seizures occur in a high proportion of patients and show a diverse pattern of both frequency and severity. The neurologic examination rarely shows a specific problem, but the EEG will often reveal a characteristic pattern consisting of nearly continuous generalized epileptic activity during slow-wave (non-REM) sleep.

Conventional antiepileptic therapy is often unsatisfactory in the Landau-Kleffner syndrome, although numerous medications have been tried. Corticosteroid therapy with prednisone has been used successfully to cause a remission in seizures; high-dose intravenous diazepam is reported to be effective in a small number of cases. Unfortunately, remission of seizures does not mean improved behavior or cognitive activity.

Rasmussen syndrome is a serious disorder of childhood that first starts with partial seizures. These are typically followed by progressive continuous partial seizures, cognitive deterioration, paralysis of one side of the body (*hemiparesis*), and shrinkage of one side of the brain (*hemiatrophy*). The seizures and brain damage remain confined to one hemisphere of the brain throughout the duration of the illness, which irreversibly culminates in the destruction of one entire cerebral hemisphere. The cause of Rasmussen syndrome is unknown. Microscopic changes in the brain resemble those seen in viral encephalitis (a viral infection of the brain), but no viral agent has ever been identified. Why only one cerebral hemisphere is affected and the other is spared is also an unsolved medical mystery. An autoimmune mechanism has been suspected but remains unproven.

The only proven effective therapy for seizures in Rasmussen syndrome is surgical removal of the affected brain hemisphere—half the brain (*hemispherectomy*). Despite the radical nature of this procedure, experience has shown that more limited procedures do not halt progression of the illness and leave the patient with persistent seizures. Most epilepsy centers perform a *functional hemispherectomy*, which surgically removes the central portion of the hemisphere and disconnects the frontal and occipital poles (Chapter 5).

Tuberous sclerosis complex (TSC) is a disorder characterized by light-colored (depigmented) skin lesions and nodular collections of abnormal cells and tissue in the brain's cerebral cortex. Apart from the brain, abnormally malformed tissue and tumors can occur in multiple organ systems, and there is a tendency for some lesions to become cancerous. Epilepsy affects 90% of patients with TSC and typically begins in the first decade of life. There is a significant incidence of infantile spasms, although partial seizures affect a much higher proportion of patients. Seizures are often *refractory* to medication and may be associated with significant developmental regression. Status epilepticus unresponsive to aggressive medical treatment has been observed as early as 2 days of age.

Infantile spasms in patients with TSC have been shown to be especially responsive to treatment with vigabatrin. The reasons for vigabatrin's good results for infantile spasms in TSC are unknown, because vigabatrin does not offer similar benefit for partial seizures due to other conditions. Conventional AEDs are often ineffective in many TSC patients with epilepsy, and surgery to remove the affected brain tissue offers a significant likelihood of seizure-freedom or improved seizure status. Despite the occurrence of multiple cortical tubers, only one is typically associated with seizure origin. Removal of the offending tuber can produce long-standing relief from seizures. Given the known natural progression of the disorder, prompt referral for surgical consideration should be carried out relatively early.

ANTIEPILEPTIC DRUGS IN CHILDREN: SPECIAL CONSIDERATIONS

Children are treated with antiepileptic medications similar to those used in adults. These effectively control most seizures in childhood, although children may not always respond to medications in the same way that adults do. For example, children typically require a higher proportional dosage compared to adults because their brain weight is proportionally larger, and children are extremely efficient at removing medications from their bodies. The liver and the kidneys, which play critical roles in eliminating medications, are at their peak performance in childhood. It may be necessary to divide daily medication into more frequent doses to maintain an even blood level.

The incidence of medication-related side effects is also different for children. Medications that are sedating in adults can have opposite effects in the very young. For example, phenobarbital produces drowsiness in older patients but results in hyperactivity in children. Phenobarbital can cause a child to be inattentive at school, and the behavioral side effects of some medications can disrupt normal social interactions like play.

Children are especially vulnerable to the side effects of certain medications and, conversely, seem resistant to others. In children, phenytoin (Dilantin) produces gum overgrowth, excessive body hair growth, and coarsening of facial features. The risk of liver toxicity by valproic acid (Depakote, Depakene) is greater in children, especially those younger than 2 years. Children are also at higher risk of serious rash from lamotrigine (Lamictal). On the other hand, children seldom experience nausea from carbamazepine (Tegretol), and it is extremely rare to encounter lowered sodium levels in children treated with carbamazepine (Tegretol) or oxcarbazepine (Trileptal). Abnormal numbness and tingling of the fingertips is reported by adult patients started on topiramate (Topamax), but this symptom is unknown in children.

Childhood is a time when healthy bones are forming. Medications can influence the metabolic aspects of bone mineralization and may adversely affect bone health by causing diminished physical activity. Some medications are more likely to produce obesity, while others lead to modest weight loss.

Some *formulations* of medication are better tolerated by children. Good-tasting liquid preparations are better tolerated in very young children, and are easily administered via a gastric tube in the disabled. Sprinkle preparations can be mixed with apple sauce, yogurt, or ice cream. Chewable and dissolvable tablets are also favored by children. Tablets with special coatings to make them less irritating to the stomach (Depakote tablets) or extended-release formulations (Tegretol-XR, Depakote-ER) may not need to be divided or broken into smaller doses. Special preparations that lack sugar are available for children whose carbohydrate intake is restricted by special treatments such as the ketogenic diet (see Chapter 6).

Because of these special concerns about AEDs in children, talk to your child's physician about the choice of medication, formulation and dosage, and potential side effects. No physician can fully predict all possible medication effects, but patients and their families should promptly communicate any unexpected or bothersome side effects.

INITIATING AND STOPPING MEDICATION

The occurrence of a single seizure does not mean that a child has epilepsy. Isolated seizures can be provoked by a wide variety of stresses such as low blood sugar (glucose) levels, abnormal sodium levels, or a febrile illness. Other children may be experiencing a benign childhood seizure disorder with a low probability of recurrence. In these situations, treatment with daily medications is rarely indicated.

The decision to start medication in children with recurrent seizures is ultimately based on the overall presentation, rather than on any single test finding. Thus, one child may have an abnormal EEG with epileptic activity, yet treatment is withheld. In contrast, another child with a different seizure type and a normal EEG may be started on medication because the seizure is typical of an epilepsy syndrome with a poor prognosis, or one that originates deep within the brain so that abnormal electrical activity is not seen on the scalp EEG.

As a rule, whenever seizures recur, the likelihood of an additional recurrence increases significantly. At this point, most physicians will start AED treatment, using the best medication for the particular seizure. The EEG helps determine whether the seizure began in one area of the brain (partial seizures) or in both cerebral hemispheres simultaneously (generalized seizure). Specific AEDs are available for each category. The advantages and liabilities of each medicine must also be considered.

The risk of immediate recurrence after a first seizure is generally low. Thus, medication should not be administered rapidly; most doctors like to "start low and go slow," beginning with a small dose and slowly increasing the dose until the seizures are controlled. This gradual escalation in dose also allows sufficient time to recognize potential side effects. Some medications, such as topiramate (Topamax), are better tolerated if the starting dose is low and the dose escalation is slow. The "start low, go slow" approach is also more likely to achieve the lowest effective AED dose.

When should medication be discontinued? Many childhood epilepsies and epilepsy syndromes are associated with a favorable prognosis characterized by seizures that do not recur after initial treatment. Children who remain seizure-free for 2 years and have a normal EEG can be safely weaned off AEDs. However, seizure-freedom after 2 years does not guarantee a reduced likelihood of seizure occurrence in certain epilepsy syndromes such as JME. Withdrawal of medications will trigger seizure recurrence in this syndrome and lead to a loss of highly prized mobility and the accompanying sense of freedom, especially if seizures restrict operation of a motor vehicle.

LEARNING AND EPILEPSY

Children with epilepsy are prone to significant trouble in school. Any underlying brain dysfunction that causes seizures may also contribute to problems with attention, memory, and learning. Studies of children with epilepsy have consistently shown a higher frequency of attention deficit-hyperactivity disorder (ADHD), autism, learning and behavioral problems, and psychiatric disorders. The success or failure in controlling the frequency and severity of seizures will also affect the way in which a child or adolescent learns. The effects of AEDs themselves can also have a significant impact on attention, memory, and other domains of cognitive function.

It is difficult to calculate the overall impact of pre-existing structural brain abnormalities on learning. Although absence of brain damage is associated with a better prognosis for intellectual functioning, some children with brain damage and cerebral palsy perform at an acceptable academic level. Many autistic children with epilepsy, cognitive, and social disabilities may have normal MRI scans. The presence of severe behavioral and cognitive abnormalities prior to seizure onset suggests that learning problems may result from underlying brain dysfunction.

Role of AEDs

Antiepileptic medications can affect alertness, concentration, memory, and learning. Certain medications have a more severe impact on learning. Barbiturates, such as phenobarbital, and the benzodiazepine class of medications, such as clonazepam (Klonopin), diazepam (Valium), lorazepam (Ativan), and clorazepate (Tranxene), impair attention at high doses and reduce school performance at moderately high doses. Barbiturates may cause depression in some patients.

In some children, AEDs can influence a child's capacity to learn. Carbamazepine (Tegretol) and oxcarbazepine (Trileptal) have not been associated with diminished school performance when administered in moderate doses, but among the newer medications, diminished word fluency is associated with topiramate (Topamax) and this effect is encountered with other AEDs as well. Irritability and anger outbursts are described in some children treated with gabapentin (Neurontin) and levetiracetam (Keppra). Behavioral changes are encountered rarely with zonisamide (Zonegran). In contrast, lamotrigine (Lamictal) has not been shown to affect intellectual or social ability in young adults.

Because all children are different, each may respond to medication differently. It's important to closely monitor your child while he is taking AEDs and report to his physician any changes in his behavior or attitude. Problems with attention, memory, and learning can be pre-existing conditions, or they can occur as treatment-related side effects. As a general rule, fewer problems are encountered when medications are started at a low dose and increased slowly. Gradual adjustment also ensures that the medication is given at the lowest effective dose. Using several AEDs at once (combination therapy) may lead to a higher risk of side effects, although recent research suggests that some combinations of newer-generation medications may work better and produce fewer side effects when used together.

Treating Other Problems

Treatment of associated problems can improve a child's learning ability and quality of life. For example, the use of stimulant medications for ADHD does not worsen seizures. Thus, a careful choice of anticonvulsant medications and an open mind toward the treatment of ADHD symptoms may have a positive effect on schooling. Some anticonvulsant medications, such as carbamazepine (Tegretol), lamotrigine (Lamictal), valproic acid (Depakote, Depakene), and occasionally gabapentin (Neurontin), have a beneficial effect on mood. The added use of medications such as fluoxetine (Prozac) or sertraline (Zoloft) may further improve depression and anxiety.

Children who are not seizure-free on medication should be considered for epilepsy surgery. Successful surgery can eliminate seizures and have a favorable effect on later cognitive functioning.

EPILEPSY SURGERY AND CHILDREN

The principles of epilepsy surgery in children are not much different from those in adults, as described in Chapter 5. The decision to refer patients for epilepsy surgery rests on the belief that medical treatment has failed. This occurs only if the physician has exercised *due diligence*—he has given the best possible medications at the high safe concentrations. However, there are few established guidelines to assist the physician's choice of medications, dosing interval, duration of treatment, monitoring of serum concentration, and withdrawal of therapy. Thus, medical treatment of seizures is still largely individualized, and there is no unique point in time when seizures can be positively identified as intractable to medication.

Two broad categories of surgical therapy exist for epilepsy—curative and palliative. *Curative surgery* eradicates seizures and the need for medication, whereas *palliative surgery* lessens seizure severity or frequency or prevents the occurrence of some seizure types. These outcome measures are similar to the goals of surgery in other conditions (e.g., for cancer surgery, complete tumor removal vs. reducing the size of a tumor).

Curative procedures involve removing a portion of the brain responsible for the epilepsy. Examples include removing a portion of a lobe of the brain, or more extensive procedures that remove multiple lobes or one cerebral hemisphere.

Because curative surgery also eliminates the psychosocial disability associated with seizures, surgery is the best hope for achieving a "normal" life, including improved schooling, greater personal independence, enhanced employment opportunities, and attainment of a driver's license. Return to a normal lifestyle rarely occurs in patients who do not achieve seizure freedom.

In some individuals, only one of several seizure types is cured by surgery, but this outcome may still be worthwhile. For example, children usually benefit from the elimination or marked reduction in the frequency of tonic or atonic seizures, due to the reduction in medical risk and injuries (e.g., fractures, lacerations from falls). Similarly, children may benefit from the stopping of complex partial seizures, and they will tolerate occasional auras without loss of consciousness. This type of palliative surgery requires a clear definition of the treatment objectives before the surgery begins, so that the results can be realistically appreciated.

Whenever surgery for epilepsy is contemplated, its risks and benefits must be weighed carefully. As in adults, the risks are usually acceptably low, with overall complications occurring in between 2% and 5% of patients. Surgical complications include stroke, hemorrhage, infection, and direct brain injury, possibly resulting in temporary or permanent neurologic deficits. Complications and death vary according to age and type of surgery; the risks of surgery appear to be slightly higher in children compared to adults and for larger procedures such as hemispherectomy.

Any risk of surgery must also be compared to the risk of continued medical treatment. At present, few studies compare the relative risks of medical versus surgical treatment. The risks associated with ongoing epilepsy and its medical treatments include death, injury, status epilepticus, possible detrimental effects of seizures, and the adverse side effects of medication. People with epilepsy have increased mortality rates compared with the general population.

FREQUENTLY ASKED QUESTIONS

Q Are seizures in the newborn harmful to its brain?

A It is now becoming clear that frequent, prolonged seizures or status epilepticus that does not respond readily to seizure medications are often indications of an underlying structural brain abnormality or birth defect, a severe lack of blood supply or oxygen to the brain, or a metabolic disorder that is preventing brain cells from obtaining energy in the normal way from food.

Prolonged seizures also cause excessive release of excitatory neurotransmitters, like glutamate and aspartate, which may make it easier for the brain to experience further seizures. In experimental animals, *recurrent* seizures can produce lasting changes that make the animal more prone to more seizures and make it harder for the animal to learn and remember. On the other hand, experimental data from immature rats found that after a *single* prolonged seizure, their brains were relatively resistant to such adverse effects. Repeated neonatal seizures and status epilepticus in experimental animals, however, are clearly detrimental to learning, memory, and activity levels. This outcome is influenced by the overlapping effects of the underlying brain abnormality, injury from various causes, and the effect of the seizures.

Q How can I tell if my newborn is experiencing a seizure?

A Seizures in the newborn may be difficult to detect. Abnormal movements or other manifestations of seizures may be subtle. Repetitive stereotyped movements should arouse concern for seizures, especially if the movements are associated with a change in behavior. Repetitive jerking of the eyes is another possible sign of possible seizures. In rare circumstances, a newborn may transiently stop breathing as the only manifestation of a seizure. If there is a suspicion that seizures are occurring, contact your doctor. It may be helpful to video-record the manifestations and show the tape to your doctor.

Q What should I do if my child experiences a convulsion during a high fever?

A Febrile seizures typically begin without warning at the onset of various childhood illnesses accompanied by fever (e.g. ear or throat infection). Because of their sudden occurrence, it is very difficult to prevent them; once the febrile seizure begins, the child should be placed on his or her side until the seizure is over. Most febrile seizures are brief and last only a few minutes. Do not place anything in the child's mouth as this may cause irritation or break teeth. Placing your finger in the child's mouth could traumatically damage your finger should the child involuntarily bite down during the seizure. If your child is prone to recurrent febrile seizures, rectal diazepam can be administered for seizures that have not stopped on their own by three minutes.

Q My child's AEDs make her irritable and hard to control. I am worried about her behavior when she starts school next year. What should I do?

A AEDs affect children differently and some produce noticeable changes in behavior and mood. These changes may become apparent immediately after starting the medicine ("idiosyncratic reaction"), or may develop when the dose is increased (toxicity). If your child's behavior changes immediately upon starting a new AED, it is best to bring this to the attention of your doctor who will probably consider stopping the AED and trying something different. If behavioral changes occur only after the AED dose is increased, your doctor may first consider lowering the dosage to eliminate the problem. This may not be possible without causing an increase in seizures. In this case, the AED should be discontinued and a different medicine tried.

Q My child's physician has tried three different medications, but nothing seems to be working. What are our options now?

A Children who continue to have seizures despite trying three different medications are considered to have intractable epilepsy. Unfortunately, the likelihood of controlling intractable seizures with a fourth or fifth AED is low. Several options exist at this point. The child may be a candidate for a specialized diet, either the ketogenic diet or a modified Atkins diet. Approximately 20–30% of children with intractable epilepsy will obtain seizure control by dietary manipulation. If dietary therapy is not an option, surgical therapy should be considered. Surgical removal of epileptic brain tissue represents an effective therapy if a well defined target can be identified. This requires a battery of tests which are typically undertaken at specialized pediatric epilepsy surgery centers. The presence of a well defined focal abnormality on the child's MRI scan often assists the surgical team in identifying the area of seizure origination. Epilepsy surgery offers the possibility or seizure freedom or improvement in a high proportion of children.

My Notes

8

EPILEPSY AND WOMEN

Concerns for Women of All Ages

Key Points

▶ Many women experience changes in seizure frequency during their menstrual cycle.

▶ Estrogen is a hormone that generally excites brain cells.

▶ Certain AEDs can lower the effectiveness of birth control pills.

▶ Polycystic ovary disease is more frequent in women with epilepsy.

▶ Somes AEDs can cause sexual problems.

▶ Over 90% of babies born to women with epilepsy are healthy.

WOMEN OF ALL AGES WITH EPILEPSY have special concerns. These concerns include the relationship of seizures and antiepileptic drugs (AEDs) with pregnancy, menstruation, birth control, sexuality, fertility, polycystic ovary syndrome, and perimenopause and menopause. This chapter explores these concerns and provides some straightforward answers to the most frequently asked questions. The first part of the chapter discusses the relationship of epilepsy to reproductive functioning, and the second part is devoted to pregnancy concerns.

EPILEPSY AND REPRODUCTIVE FUNCTIONING IN WOMEN

Onset of Seizures at Puberty and Relationship to Hormonal Changes

Several types of seizure disorders often begin in the early teenage years, when menstrual periods also begin for many young women. The types of seizure disorders that start at this age include juvenile myoclonic epilepsy (JME) and juvenile absence epilepsy (JAE).

Although JME is more common in females than in males, no clear scientific evidence indicates that gender-related reproductive *hormones*—such as testosterone, estrogen, or progesterone—are associated with the timing of the onset of these seizure types for either young women or men.

The Relationship of the Menstrual Cycle and Seizures

Approximately one-third of women with epilepsy can have a near doubling of the number of seizures at specific times of the month, in relation to their menstrual cycle. The term used for seizures that occur in relation to the menstrual cycle is *catamenial epilepsy*. Catamenial epilepsy refers only to the timing of the seizures and not to a specific seizure type. In fact, catamenial epilepsy can occur with all seizure types, including simple partial, complex partial, or generalized seizures. The most frequent time at which a seizure flare-up (or *exacerbation*) occurs for women with catamenial seizures is during the few days prior to menstrual bleeding and including the first day of menses. The second most common time of the month when seizures tend to exacerbate is at ovulation, in the middle of the menstrual cycle. The third most frequent pattern of seizure exacerbation is during the entire 2 weeks prior to menses, including the time of ovulation and continuing until menstrual onset.

The times of seizure worsening for women of reproductive age with epilepsy are related to normal hormonal changes throughout the month. One of the main female reproductive hormones, estrogen, is active in and has various functions in the brain. These functions include regulating reproductive and sexual activity and maintaining the interconnectedness of brain cells. Estrogen is a hormone that generally excites brain activity, and therefore is more seizure-promoting than seizure-preventing. On the other hand, the other main reproductive hormone for women, progesterone, tends to be calming and sedating. Progesterone, therefore, actually helps to inhibit brain activity in general and can inhibit seizure activity as well.

The timing of seizure occurrence in relationship to the menstrual cycle is probably related to the normal up and down cycle of these two hormones throughout the month. For example, progesterone levels decline dramatically just before menstrual onset, which correlates with what can be called premenstrual "progesterone withdrawal." This progesterone withdrawal is thought to make women with epilepsy more likely to have seizures in the days just before menses and on the first day. On the other hand, estrogen levels rise and reach a peak just before ovulation at the middle of the menstrual cycle. This estrogen peak is thought to influence the occurrence of seizures at mid-cycle, when ovulation occurs.

Another time of the month when women with epilepsy are susceptible to seizures is during the 2 weeks prior to menses, also called the *luteal phase*. This exacerbation in seizure activity is likely related to hormonal changes during those months when ovulation does not occur. Women with epilepsy tend to frequently have menstrual cycles in which they do not ovulate, meaning that an egg is not released from the ovary for that month, and therefore pregnancy cannot occur. In women without epilepsy, this *anovulatory* cycle occurs normally about once per year. Women with epilepsy have anovulatory cycles two to three times per year. Levels of the naturally occurring anti-seizure hormone progesterone are especially low during anovulatory cycles, which creates another situation in which seizures are more likely to occur in women with epilepsy.

Treatment of Seizure Worsening in Relationship to the Menstrual Cycle

No medication is specifically proven to help reduce catamenial seizure exacerbations. This is probably the main reason why women with epilepsy feel that their doctors do not adequately discuss the situation when they report that their seizures are occurring in relationship to menstruation. Unfortunately, sometimes when a physician cannot easily offer a treatment for a medical problem, it becomes frustrating for both the physician and the patient. Therefore, although your doctor may seem to be minimizing the problem, this not necessarily the case. Some reasonable interventions for catamenial seizure worsening are discussed next.

Natural Progesterone

Since the progesterone produced by the body has antiseizure properties, it has been used to prevent catamenial seizure exacerbations. Natural progesterone can be given in a pill (Prometrium) or lozenge form, and it is also available as a cream. It is generally used for obstetric and gynecologic purposes, but the use of natural progesterone to treat catamenial seizures is currently being investigated by the National Institutes of Health at many sites around the United States. Natural progesterone has been prescribed for catamenial seizure exacerbations during the 2 weeks prior to menses, continuing through the first day of menstrual bleeding. Although natural progesterone is the same hormone naturally produced by your body, side effects can occur. These are generally mild and include sedation, depressed mood, breast tenderness, and vaginal spotting. Synthetic progesterone, used in most birth control pills and in hormone replacement therapy, does not prevent seizure activity in the same way as natural progesterone since it is not active in the same brain areas.

Increased Doses of AEDs

Perhaps the most common approach to treating catamenial seizure exacerbations is to slightly increase the dose of the AEDs already being taken, during vulnerable times of the month. Usually, one medication is increased slightly for several days premenstrually. For most AEDs, an increase of 10% to 25% of the total daily dose for several days will not cause significant problems, such as side effects or drug interactions. However, some medications, such as phenytoin, may cause *toxicity* even with a small dose increase; any premenstrual adjustment in medication should be carefully considered and discussed with your neurologist.

Acetazolamide (Diamox)

Acetazolamide (Diamox) has been also used premenstrually to prevent catamenial seizure worsening. This treatment has been used for decades, but has never been proven to actually reduce seizure occurrence. Many women have reported benefit from using acetazolamide for the first few months of treatment, but then report that the effect seems to "wear off." Acetazolamide is a mild diuretic and is usually used for the treatment of glaucoma. Its mechanism of action in preventing seizures is unknown.

Use of Hormonal Birth Control for Women with Epilepsy

Hormonal birth control methods can be used safely and effectively for women with epilepsy. It has been reported that oral contraceptive pills ("the pill") have a higher failure rate—that is, are associated with more unplanned pregnancies—when women are taking certain AEDs. The failure rate of the oral contraceptive pill (getting pregnant!) for women with epilepsy taking those AEDs listed in Table 8.1 is reported to be around 6% per year. However, women using oral contraceptive pills and not taking AEDs can have a failure rate of 2% to 7% per year, and these pregnancies are most often due to missing doses of the oral contraceptives. Therefore, even with this slightly increased rate of birth control failure with oral contraceptive pills while taking AEDs, the chance of preventing pregnancy (around 94%) is better than with most other commonly used birth control methods, such as condoms or diaphragm use, and is certainly better than the "rhythm method."

Only some of the AEDs lower the effectiveness of birth control pills (Table 8.1). This happens because these particular AEDs lower the blood (or serum) level of the hormones released from the oral contraceptive pills, making them less effective. To counteract this effect, the American

TABLE 8.1
Antiepileptic Medications and Oral Contraceptives

Should be used with higher dose oral contraceptives	May be used with any oral contraceptives	Level of antiseizure medication is decreased by oral contraceptive
Phenytoin (Phenytoin)	Zonisamide (Zonegran)	Lamotrigine (Lamictal)
Primidone (Mysoline)	Valproate (Depakote)	
Carbamazepine (Tegretol, Carbatrol)	Tiagabine (Gabitril)	
Topiramate (Topamax)	Levetiracetam (Keppra)	
Oxcarbazepine (Trileptal)	Ethosuximide (Zarontin)	
Felbamate (Felbatol)	Lacosamide (Vimpat)	
Rufinamide (Banzel)		

Academy of Neurology has recommended that women with epilepsy use an oral contraceptive pill that contains a high dose of estrogen, preferably 50 micrograms (µg). You should discuss this with your gynecologist and obtain an appropriate prescription. If you use Depo-Provera for birth control, more frequent injections, at every 10 weeks instead of every 12 weeks, is recommended. Recommendations for altering the use of other hormonal birth control methods are not available. The most effective way of preventing pregnancy while using hormonal contraception for women with epilepsy is to use it in combination with another method, such as a diaphragm or a condom. In Table 8.1, the interactions between AEDs and hormonal contraceptives are shown in using the generic and brand names (in parentheses). Higher-dose oral contraceptives are listed in Table 8.2.

Some AEDs have no interactions with birth control pills. Only one AED, lamotrigine, is known to have its own level decreased by oral contraceptives. Therefore, if you take lamotrigine, you may need to adjust your dose when you start using a hormonal contraceptive, because you may be at risk for seizure occurrence as your lamotrigine level goes down.

Polycystic Ovary Syndrome and Epilepsy

Polycystic ovary syndrome (PCOS) occurs in about 5% of women in general and in about 10% of women with epilepsy, no matter which AED they are taking. This *syndrome* is made up of several disorders, including two of these three: multiple cysts on the ovaries, high male hormone levels, or physical signs of high male hormone levels, such as excessive facial hair and acne. Therefore, ovarian cysts are not a required feature to make the diagnosis of PCOS. Weight gain

TABLE 8.2
Oral contraceptives considered to be higher dose and should be used with antiseizure medications in the first column of Table 8.1

Demulen 1/50	Ogestrel
Necon 1/35	Ortho-Novum 1/35
Necon 1/50	Ortho-Novum 1/50
Norinyl 1+35	Ovcon 50
Norinyl 1+50	Ovral-28
Nortrel 1/35	Zovia 1/50E

(Note: 50 refers to 50 µg of estrogen)

and inability to lose weight is often part of the illness, as are irregular menstrual periods and frequent periods during which ovulation does not occur. Therefore, often the most serious consequence of having PCOS is the inability to get pregnant readily, and this syndrome is a major cause of infertility.

The cause of PCOS is unknown. The cause may be related to abnormal glucose metabolism in the body. In women with epilepsy, it is believed that seizure activity in the brain—and even the small electrical discharges that occur without seizures (*interictal* spikes on EEG)—may alter the normal reproductive hormone secretion from nearby structures in the brain, such as the hypothalamus and pituitary. This alteration in normal hormonal secretion in women with epilepsy could be the cause or at least contribute to the onset of PCOS.

Polycystic Ovary Syndrome and Valproate

Valproate (Depakote, Depakote ER, Depakene) causes features of PCOS in some women, including weight gain, mild increases in male hormone levels, and irregular menstrual periods with a decreased rate of ovulation. It is unclear if valproate causes PCOS itself or if valproate has side effects that fit with PCOS.

Monitoring for PCOS in Women with Epilepsy

Keep track of the regularity of your menstrual periods and report on this to your doctor, including your neurologist. You should also monitor weight changes and notice if weight gain occurs with the use of any AEDs, such as valproate. Gabapentin and carbamazepine can also cause weight gain. Report weight changes, difficulty getting pregnant, and the occurrence of acne or hair changes to your physician as well. If these problems are occurring, either in relation to valproate use or without its use, a consultation with a gynecologist or reproductive endocrinologist should be planned.

Keep in mind that, although physicians are trained to take care of patients in their entirety, your neurologist may be more focused on seizures, medication side effects, and neurologic complaints. Therefore, you should make your neurologists aware when these symptoms of reproductive dysfunction occur, so she can make an appropriate referral for evaluation and treatment. If valproate is being used as an antiseizure treatment, your neurologist may consider changing it to another medication, depending on how well valproate has worked for you and how difficult the seizures are to control. Treatments for PCOS are varied and are specific for each patient. They can include progesterone, weight management, or insulin use. Women with PCOS who have fertility problems may become pregnant with treatment of the syndrome, so seeking treatment is often well worth the effort.

Sexual Functioning in Women with Epilepsy

The majority of women with epilepsy report normal satisfaction with their sexual lives. However, a larger-than-expected number of women with epilepsy report very little interest in sex. The exact reasons for this are unclear, and are possibly related to anxiety about having a seizure in an intimate situation, for example. Women with epilepsy do report more anxiety about sexual situations than expected. Further, there is some evidence that the physical sexual response, such as vaginal lubrication, is decreased in women with epilepsy, but it is not known whether this is due to the epilepsy itself or to AED.

Some AEDs have a known risk of causing problems with sexuality. These are primarily the sedative medications, phenobarbital and primidone. Sexual side effects have been reported with many of the AEDs however, including phenytoin, carbamazepine, valproate, and gabapentin. The cause of sexual side effects for persons with epilepsy may be related to subtle effects of the AEDs on reproductive hormone levels, including the main hormone associated with sexual interest, testosterone. However, a direct effect of these medications on brain chemicals that regulate sexual activity may also be occurring.

Most women with epilepsy have normal sexual lives, with the usual difficulties that many people face in a busy, stressful world. If sexuality is a problem—either interest in sex (libido) or the ability to achieve orgasm (sexual functioning)—you should not hesitate to discuss this with your neurologist. Your neurologist may consider changing your AED, if the problem occurred in association with a specific medication, or she may refer you to a gynecologist or sexual therapist as well. Treatments such as sildenafil (Viagra) or testosterone replacement have not yet been proven effective or completely safe for women.

Infertility and Epilepsy

In several surveys, women with epilepsy were found to have lower rates of having children than both their own siblings and the general population. This does not necessarily mean that women with epilepsy are *infertile*, which means a biologic inability to become pregnant. It may be that women with epilepsy have fewer children because they choose not to, because of their epilepsy and the medications they must take. Although choice is likely a factor, some degree of biologic infertility may also play a part, since it is clear that women with epilepsy have more menstrual periods during which they don't ovulate and therefore cannot get pregnant for that month. Other reproductive abnormalities, such as the presence of PCOS, may also contribute to infertility. No specific AED has been associated with infertility, however.

If you are having difficulty getting pregnant after trying for more than 6 months, seek guidance from your gynecologist regarding an infertility evaluation.

Although current information indicates that women with well-controlled epilepsy have only slightly increased risks for additional problems associated with pregnancy and birth outcomes, some concern still exists on the part of patients and even physicians regarding pregnancy and epilepsy.

Epilepsy during Perimenopause and Menopause

Perimenopause, when women begin to have irregular menses and hot flashes, may be a time of risk for more seizures. The hormonal changes of early perimenopause, when a woman's estrogen levels are generally higher than her progesterone levels, may explain why this is a vulnerable time for women with epilepsy. However, the good news is that women with epilepsy may have a decrease in their seizures when they complete menopause and become postmenopausal. Both of these effects occur more prominently when women have had a catamenial seizure pattern during their reproductive years, which suggests that these women in particular are sensitive to hormonal fluctuations. An increase in seizure activity during perimenopause should be carefully evaluated and treated with an adjustment in antiseizure treatments.

Women with epilepsy, particularly those who have had frequent seizures during their lifetime, may experience an earlier-than-expected menopause. The usual age at which menstruation ceases is around 50 to 51 years. Menstruation may cease slightly sooner in women with frequent seizure, around age 46 to 47 years. The cause of this is unknown, but may be due to effects of seizures on those parts of the brain that regulate reproductive functioning.

The risks of long-term hormone replacement therapy (HRT) for women in general include a small increased risk of breast cancer and of cardiovascular disease and stroke. Therefore, the use of the most common type of HRT, conjugated equine estrogen combined with medroxyprogesterone acetate (CEE/MPA or Prempro), has been drastically reduced. However, severe and disabling hot flashes during perimenopause and postmenopausally can disrupt sleep, and, in women with epilepsy, sleep deprivation can increase the risk of seizures. Therefore, some women absolutely need to take hormone replacement for a short period so that they don't become too sleep-deprived and are able to function normally on a daily basis.

HRT may increase seizure frequency. Some menopausal women with epilepsy have reported this problem with the use of CEE/MPA. If you need to use short-term hormone replacement to manage hot flashes, you should discuss an appropriate regimen and duration of treatment with your gynecologist. Using estradiol combined with natural progesterone as short-term HRT may be an alternative choice, since natural progesterone may have an anti-seizure effect.

Pregnancy for Women with Epilepsy

Epilepsy is the most common neurologic disorder that requires continuous treatment during pregnancy. Although there are risks due to seizures and seizure medications during pregnancy, over 90% of babies born to women with epilepsy will be healthy. Seizure control is essential, and most women must be maintained on a seizure medication (anticonvulsant) during pregnancy. The emphasis is how to minimize the risks of these medications to a level that is no different from the risks of a pregnancy in a woman on no medications and with no underlying illness (the general population). In the general population, a 1.6% to 3.2% rate of birth defects is possible in newborns. In infants born to women with epilepsy on seizure medications, the birth defect rate is about twice that (4%–7%).

Ideally, the seizure medications and vitamin supplementation you take should be reviewed prior to pregnancy to minimize risks to the developing fetus. You should take extra folic acid to reduce the risk of birth defects. Many doctors recommend that all women get into the habit of taking supplemental folic acid once they reach their reproductive years. If possible, your medications should be reduced to just one AED (*monotherapy*). (Some monotherapy regimens may be more or less dangerous during pregnancy.) All this must be considered against the backdrop of which medications you must have to control your seizures.

The best path to a healthy pregnancy is a planned pregnancy with an open dialogue with the doctor prescribing your seizure medications and your obstetrician, a review of the latest findings about specific seizure medications during pregnancy, and use of supplemental folic acid and/or prenatal vitamins. The pregnancy checklist in Figure 8.1 provides a quick and easy guide for women on seizure medications.

Features of the Fetal Anticonvulsant Syndrome

Birth defects that require surgery or can significantly affect the child's life are called *major malformations*. Unfortunately, major malformations are part of the *fetal anticonvulsant syndrome* (FAS), a group of disorders that may occur when a pregnant women takes certain antiepileptic medications. Other features of FAS include minor *anomalies*, *intrauterine growth retardation*, cognitive dysfunction, *microcephaly*, and an increased chance of early death.

FIGURE 8.1
Checklist for women with epilepsy planning or during a pregnancy.

Pre-Conception (prior to pregnancy)

▶ You should be taking the following medications daily, as suggested by your doctor, in addition to your seizure medication(s):
1. Multivitamins or prenatal vitamins
2. Folic acid 0.4–5 mg

▶ Discuss with your doctor that you are planning a pregnancy and want to transition to the best medication regimen for the safety of you and your developing child.

▶ Additional Resources: Epilepsy Foundation Brochures, and web sites:
http://www.efa.org
http://www.massgeneral.org/aed

Pregnancy

▶ For the duration of your pregnancy, you should be taking the following medications daily, as prescribed by your doctor:
1. Multivitamins or prenatal vitamins
2. Folic acid 0.4–5 mg

▶ The level of medication in your blood may decrease during pregnancy.

▶ It is recommended that you discuss with your doctor regular monitoring of your drug levels during pregnancy and after childbirth.

▶ The dose of your seizure medications may be changed based upon the results of your lab tests, worsening of seizures, or because of side effects of the medication.

▶ It is very important not to miss doses. If you have problems with vomiting within 30 minutes of taking your seizure medication, you should repeat the dose.

▶ Your doctor will schedule you for a maternal alpha-fetoprotein and/or "triple screen" at 15–22 weeks gestation.

▶ A detailed, structural (level II) ultrasound will be ordered at 16–20 weeks of gestation. This will often be performed by a perinatologist.

▶ Vitamin K (10 mg daily) may be prescribed beginning at 36 weeks of gestation until delivery to prevent bleeding disorders in the infant.

FIGURE 8.1 (CONTINUED)
Checklist for women with epilepsy planning or during a pregnancy.

▶   Identify a pediatrician at least 1 month prior to your due date and discuss your plans for breast-feeding.

▶   You should discuss a birth plan with your obstetrician and your doctor who is prescribing your seizure medication.

Day of Delivery

▶   Take a copy of your birth plan to the hospital. Notify your seizure doctor of your delivery to help manage any complications of changes in your seizures or in your medication levels.

▶   Take your seizure medications as directed. Do not miss any in the hospital during labor, delivery, and postpartum.

▶   Bring an extra supply of your seizure medication with you to the hospital.

▶   Following delivery, you may be asked to decrease your antiseizure medication.

Please be aware of side effects or other possible complications associated with seizure medications and pregnancy. If you are feeling different from usual, inform your doctor.

If your seizures get worse during your pregnancy, call your doctor. If you have a convulsive seizure, contact your obstetrician—you may need to go to the Emergency Room.

Minor Anomalies

Minor anomalies are not of significant concern as they do not create a threat to the health of the baby. However, sometimes they may signal more concerning features of FAS, such as major malformations or developmental delay. Minor anomalies occur in 6% to 20% of infants born to women with epilepsy, a rate approximately 2.5 times higher than in the general population.

Major Malformations

Major malformations are abnormalities occurring in an essential anatomic structure, such as the face, mouth, or internal organs. These abnormalities interfere significantly with the baby's health and may require major treatment, such as surgery. The major malformations (Table 8.3) most commonly associated with antiseizure medication exposure include congenital heart defects, cleft lip or cleft palate, defects of the kidney and genital structures, and *neural tube defects* of the lower spine (often, *spina bifida*).

TABLE 8.3
Major malformations in infants of women with epilepsy

	General population	Infants of women with epilepsy
Congenital heart	0.5%	1.5–2%
Cleft lip/palate	0.15%	1.4%
Neural tube defect	0.06%	1–3.8% (VPA)
		0.5–1% (CBZ)
Urogenital defects	0.7%	1.7%

The neural tube of the spine closes during the third and fourth weeks of pregnancy to form the normal, healthy spinal column. If the neural tube does not close properly, the resulting spina bifida can cause weakness in the baby's legs and a possible lack of control over the bladder and bowels. Folic acid supplementation is the single most important thing you can do to prevent neural tube defects in your child. Because neural tube defects occur so early in pregnancy, it's important to remember that, by the time you realize you are pregnant, it may be too late to start taking supplements or adjusting your medications. This is why it is so important that *all* pregnancies in women with epilepsy be *planned pregnancies*.

High-Risk Seizure Medications

FAS has been described in association with virtually all seizure medications. The risk for major malformations is consistently higher for women on multiple AEDs (*polytherapy*) compared to women on just one seizure medication (monotherapy). In one study, the rate of major malformations increased to 25% for those women on four or more seizure medications Most physicians agree that monotherapy is preferred to polytherapy during pregnancy. The switch to monotherapy should be made during the preconception planning phase.

Recent information from pregnancy registries has helped to define risks of certain seizure medications when used alone as monotherapy. Studies by the Antiepileptic Drug Pregnancy Registry (Figure 8.2, page 154) show that, of infants born to women receiving phenobarbital as their only seizure medication, 6.5% had major malformations. For women on valproic acid monotherapy, major malformations occurred in 10.7% of their infants. This rate is four times higher that for any other seizure medication.

Little is known about the effects of the newer seizure medications (those introduced since 1990) on pregnancy. The exception to this is lamotrigine (Lamictal). The general opinion is that lamotrigine is fairly safe to take during pregnancy, with a reported rate of major malformations of between 2% and 3%. Studies are being done on the safe use of oxcarbazepine (Trileptal) during pregnancy.

If you become pregnant while taking an antiepileptic medication, you can participate in the effort to learn about the effects of these medications on pregnancy. Your participation in the North American Pregnancy Registry is greatly appreciated by everyone in the epilepsy community—other women with epilepsy, physicians, and research scientists. See Figure 8.2, page 154, for details about the North American Pregnancy Registry and how to participate.

Prenatal Screening

If you are on a seizure medication during pregnancy, your doctor may recommend that you undergo prenatal screening to detect any fetal major malformations. Although only a fraction of women may consider therapeutic abortions, the prenatal diagnosis of a heart malformation or a neural tube defect allows your pregnancy care team to make special plans for labor, delivery, and neonatal care. Surgery may be indicated immediately after birth, and surgery prior to birth is becoming more possible for some heart defects. See the pregnancy checklist in Figure 8.1 for a list of the recommended tests.

Intrauterine Growth Retardation

Intrauterine growth retardation, resulting in a low birth weight of less than 5.5 pounds, occurs in 7% to 10% of infants born to women with epilepsy. If your weight gain or size does not seem appropriate, additional ultrasounds may be repeated to assess fetal size and the condition of the amniotic fluid.

Neurodevelopmental Outcome

The children born to some women with epilepsy may be at risk for developmental delay or lower verbal abilities. A variety of factors may contribute to this, including five or more convulsive (generalized *tonic–clonic*) seizures during pregnancy and some AEDs. Phenobarbital and valproic acid (Depakote) seem to be the most likely medications to cause these problems in the unborn fetus. If the mother is on polytherapy, the risk to the fetus appears to be increased even further. Exposure during the third trimester may be the most detrimental.

Microcephaly

Microcephaly has been associated with AED use during pregnancy. The risk for small head circumference is increased in women using polytherapy, phenobarbital, and primidone (Mysoline).

YOUR CHILD'S RISK FOR EPILEPSY

Children of women with epilepsy are at slightly higher risk (about three times) of developing epilepsy at some point in their lifetime than are children without a family history of epilepsy. Overall, children of fathers with epilepsy do not demonstrate this same increased risk.

SEIZURES DURING PREGNANCY

The effect of pregnancy on seizure frequency is variable and unpredictable between patients. According to recent studies, approximately 25% of patients will have an increase in their seizures during pregnancy, 15% will see a decrease in seizures, and 60% will experience no significant change. Pregnancy is associated with several physiologic and psychologic changes that can alter seizure frequency, including changes in sex hormone levels, changes in the way your body *metabolizes* your AEDs, changes in sleep patterns, and new stresses.

Risk of Seizures to the Fetus

During pregnancy, the risk of seizures to your developing baby is of primary importance. Convulsive (generalized tonic-clonic) seizures in the mother can cause low oxygen levels in the fetus and signs of fetal distress. These seizures may even cause miscarriage or *spontaneous abortion*. Seizures that may cause you to fall can result in rupture of the membranes protecting the fetus, premature labor, and even fetal death. During pregnancy, you must take extra steps to make sure both you and your developing baby are protected from falls and other injuries, even apparently minor ones.

Risk of Seizure Medications to the Fetus

Many women neglect to take their AEDs during pregnancy, mostly because of fear that any drugs they take will harm their baby. However, you and your physician must balance the risk of possible seizures with the risk of your medications. In most cases, having a seizure while pregnant puts your baby at more risk of harm than does taking your AEDs.

The management of AEDs during pregnancy can be complex. The blood levels of all AEDs decrease during pregnancy due to changes in your body's composition and metabolism. Some medications, such as lamotrigine (Lamictal), are particularly prone to decreased levels in the bloodstream during pregnancy because of changes in how your body metabolizes the drugs. Most of these changes gradually normalize over the first few weeks to months after your baby is born.

NEONATAL VITAMIN K DEFICIENCY

Vitamin K deficiency in the newborn can cause serious bleeding. Because many AEDs can cause vitamin K deficiencies in the developing fetus, your doctor may prescribe extra vitamin K for you to take beginning in the last month of pregnancy. (Your baby will also receive a shot of vitamin K at birth, which is standard procedure for all babies born in the United States.)

LABOR AND DELIVERY

The majority of women with epilepsy will have a safe vaginal delivery without having a seizure. Having epilepsy and taking AEDs do not limit your options concerning what type of delivery you choose or whether you choose to use pain medication during delivery. The exception to this is meperidine (Demerol); meperidine should be avoided because of its potential to lower your seizure threshold. Only a small fraction of women with epilepsy will have seizures during labor or in the first few days after delivery. However, seizure recurrence may be more likely in women with primary generalized epilepsy, possibly due to their sensitivity to sleep disruption—and a new baby may mean some sleepless nights!

POSTPARTUM CARE

Most women with epilepsy can successfully breast-feed their babies without complications. The concentrations of most seizure medications are considerably less in breast milk than what the fetus was exposed to while in the womb. The benefits to your baby of breast-feeding far outweigh the small risk of side-effects from your seizure medications. However, you should watch for signs of increased drowsiness in your baby, to the degree that interferes with feeding. Your physician will also track your baby's growth and development, to ensure that your AEDs are not causing any problems.

The newborn period, with its inevitable sleep-disruption, can be a time of seizure worsening and may even provoke seizure recurrence for women with previously controlled seizures. Extra precautions should be taken during this time. If your seizures make you likely to drop objects, as occurs with myoclonic seizures or many complex partial seizures, use a harness when carrying your baby. If you are likely to fall during a seizure, then using a stroller—even in the house—is an even better option.

Changing time is best done on the floor, rather than on an elevated changing table. Bathing should never be performed alone, as a brief lapse in attention can result in a fatal drowning. The important role that sleep deprivation plays in worsening seizures must be considered. If you are breast-feeding, sleep deprivation may be unavoidable. Consider having other adults share the burden of night-time feedings through the use of formula or harvested breast-milk, and you should attempt to make up any missed sleep during your baby's daytime naps.

Women with epilepsy on seizure medications do have increased risks for complications, but these risks can be considerably reduced through effective planning prior to pregnancy and careful management during pregnancy and the postpartum period.

FIGURE 8.2
Antiepileptic Drug Pregnancy Registry Massachusetts General Hospital, Harvard Medical School

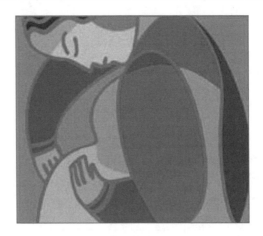

If you are pregnant, and take antiepileptic drugs (ANTISEIZURE MEDICATIONS), please call TOLL FREE (888) 233-2334 to register with the ANTISEIZURE MEDICATIONS Pregnancy Registry

What is the purpose of the Registry?
At present, we lack complete information about the relative safety of specific antiepileptic drugs (AEDs) during pregnancy. The Registry enrolls women over the telephone who are pregnant and taking seizure medications to find the answers. As more women register and report the outcome of their pregnancy, the researchers of this registry will be able to identify the safest medications for seizures during pregnancy.

When should I call the Registry?
As early in your pregnancy as possible. It is best to enroll during your 1st trimester, but you can still participate if you are already in your 2nd or 3rd trimester.

How do I register? By calling toll free (888) 233-2334.

There are only three telephone interviews:

1. The first call is the longest and can take up to 12 minutes.

2. The registry will call you when you are 7 months pregnant (5-minute call).

3. The registry will call you again after your baby is born (5-minute call).

Your identity will remain confidential!

More information can be found at http://www.massgeneral.org/antiseizure medications/

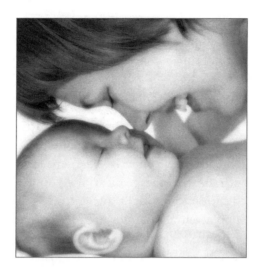

FREQUENTLY ASKED QUESTIONS

Q How can pregnancy affect my seizures?

A Most women will not see a change in their seizures. However, one-quarter to one-third of women with epilepsy will have an increase in seizure activity during their pregnancy. It is important to take your medication as prescribed by your doctor and not miss any doses. Even if you take all your doses of medication during pregnancy, the concentrations of seizure medications in your bloodstream may change or decrease, putting you at greater risk for seizures. Your physician may need to check blood levels of your medication more often, and she may need to adjust your dose. The first 2 months after delivery are another important time when your hormones and your body chemistry may change, affecting levels of your seizure medication. Check with your doctor or nurse about extra lab work that may be necessary.

Q I have received conflicting information about the safety of medications during pregnancy and breast-feeding. What should I believe?

A This is a tough question. The risks of seizure medications during pregnancy and breast-feeding are often exaggerated, even by physicians. The Internet is a great source of information, but not all the information is reviewed for scientific accuracy. Similarly, your pharmacist can provide you the information from the *Physicians Desk Reference* (PDR). The PDR is essentially a compiled set of package inserts that represents limited information in many cases. Many articles and books are typically 1 or 2 years behind the available research information. The references on the web sites listed in Figure 8.2 include some of the most reputable and current sources of information. Please remember that none of these sources takes into account your individual situation and the severity of your illness. It is important that you discuss this with your doctor prescribing your seizure medication.

Q I just found out that I am pregnant, and I am taking medications, what should I do?

A First, don't panic! The risks of seizure medications are relatively modest, and exposure has already occurred. If you were to stop your medication(s) suddenly, your seizures could be longer and more severe than any that you have experienced before. This puts you and your pregnancy at much higher risk than the medications you are on. Do let your doctor prescribing your seizure medication know right away, to make sure your dose, your medication regimen, and your supplemental vitamins are ideal for pregnancy. Also, establish care by an obstetrician early in your pregnancy for close follow-up during pregnancy, including planning for a detailed, structural ultrasound. Some obstetricians may choose to perform ultrasounds more frequently than once.

Q Should I stop my antiepileptic medication before I get pregnant?

A This is a complicated decision. Pregnancy without AEDs may lessen some of the possible risks to the baby in very specific cases. Discuss with your doctor whether you are a candidate to come off medications if you have not had seizures for several years. You will also need to have an epilepsy syndrome that is likely to remit. However, most adult women cannot come off seizure medications safely, and the danger of seizures to both the mother and the child is a serious one. Seizures can result in falls or in lack of oxygen for the baby. They can increase the risk of miscarriage or stillbirths. For most women with epilepsy, staying on medication poses less risk to their own health and the health of their babies than discontinuing medication. In most cases, a single medication at the lowest possible dose that provides seizure control is the best option.

Q I think my menstrual cycle affects my seizures. Is this possible, or am I imagining it?

A Yes, it is possible, and you are not imagining it. The hormonal changes of estrogen and progesterone throughout the month can influence seizure occurrence. This does not mean that women who do not have epilepsy can get seizures from menstrual cycling. However, for women with epilepsy, hormonal changes can influence seizure occurrence. Approximately one-third of women with epilepsy can have a near doubling of the number of seizures at specific times of the month, in relationship to their menstrual cycle. The term used for seizures that occur in relationship to the menstrual cycle is *catamenial epilepsy*.

Q Will my seizures change during perimenopause, menopause, and postmenopause?

A There is some suggestion that *perimenopause*, when women begin to have irregular menses and hot flashes, may be a time of risk for more seizures. The hormonal changes of early perimenopause, when the estrogen levels are generally higher than the progesterone levels, may explain why this is a vulnerable time for women with epilepsy. However, the good news is that women with epilepsy may have a decrease in their seizures when they complete menopause and become postmenopausal. Both of these effects occur more prominently when women have had a catamenial seizure pattern during their reproductive years, and suggest that these women are particularly sensitive to hormonal fluctuations. An increase in seizure activity during perimenopause should be carefully evaluated and treated with an adjustment in antiseizure treatments.

My Notes

_____

_____

_____

_____

_____

_____

_____

9

EPILEPSY IN SPECIAL POPULATIONS

Elderly, Brain Tumors and Bone Health

Key Points

▶ Fainting is the most frequent cause of loss of consciousness in a person, especially in the elderly.

▶ Strokes are the most common cause of new-onset seizures in the elderly, accounting for about 40% to 50% of new-onset epilepsy in this age group.

▶ Selecting an AED for an elderly patient is even more important than for a child since life-long treatment may be needed.

▶ Seizures are a common and sometimes devastating complication of brain tumors, and meticulous attention to their diagnosis and treatment is critical.

▶ Several older AEDs, such as carbamazepine, phenobarbital, phenytoin, and primidone, are most commonly associated with osteoporosis.

THIS CHAPTER ADDRESSES a few special conditions and situations, such as seizures in the elderly, special problems in patients with brain tumors, and the effects of some antiepileptic drugs (AEDs) on bone health.

SEIZURES AND EPILEPSY IN THE ELDERLY

As life expectancy continues to increase, it is harder and harder to define who is an elder. Two hundred years ago, a 40-year-old was considered old; nowadays, a 60-year-old is still looked upon as relatively young (Figure 9.1). For most working definitions, *elderly* is someone *older than 65 years*. As we get older, the possibility of having seizures increases with each passing decade. Those older than 85 have more than three times the chance for having a seizure than do 70-year-olds. Because this is the most rapidly growing segment of our population, new-onset epilepsy in the elderly is a very important issue. It is also important because the elderly react differently to drugs used to treat seizures, and the causes of seizures and epilepsy in the elderly are different from those in children and young adults.

Seizures and Epilepsy Types in the Elderly

As with any person experiencing a seizure, the first questions that should be addressed are whether the patient indeed had an epileptic seizure and, if so, whether the seizure was provoked. As we have seen in other chapters, it is important to be sure that a seizure is not confused with fainting or *syncope*. Fainting is the most frequent cause of loss of consciousness in a person, especially in the elderly. Many individuals in this age group have conditions affecting the heart or blood pressure and thus are prone to faint. True seizures however can also be caused by chemical

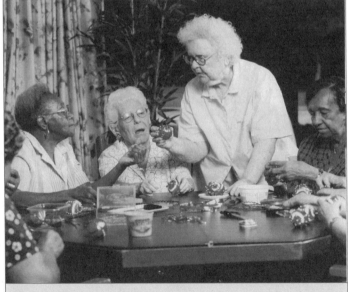

FIGURE 9.1
Seizures in the elderly are becoming more frequent.

disturbances (e.g., low blood sugar or low salt), certain medications, medication withdrawal (e.g., Valium), or substance abuse (e.g., alcohol, drugs). Although these are truly seizures, they typically do not require AED treatment and are considered *provoked* seizures.

If a seizure is unprovoked, and it is clear that we are dealing with epilepsy, then it's important to classify the seizure type to determine what type of treatment is needed. As we know by now, epileptic seizures can be *idiopathic* (with an unknown cause, although genetics are suspected in many idiopathic cases), *symptomatic*, or *cryptogenic*. Symptomatic seizures have an identified or suspected cause, such as a tumor or stroke. The cause may be identified by *imaging* (brain scans), such as magnetic resonance imaging (MRI) or computed tomography (CT). Cryptogenic seizures have a suspected cause that cannot be definitively identified (i.e., imaging is inconclusive). Most elderly patients with new-onset epilepsy have either cryptogenic or symptomatic seizures. However, in the largest study of the elderly (the Veterans Administration Cooperative Study), 25% of the patients had seizures of unknown—idiopathic—cause.

Generalized seizures most often have a genetic cause and start before age 18 years. Therefore, new-onset seizures in the elderly are *partial seizures*, either *simple* or *complex*, with possible convulsions. This is the case for most people in this group; most apparent new-onset *absence seizures* in the elderly (episodes of staring and loss of attention) are actually complex partial seizures. Finding the correct diagnosis can be a challenging problem.

Causes of Epilepsy in the Elderly

Strokes are the most common cause of new-onset seizures in the elderly, accounting for about 40% to 50% of new-onset epilepsy in this age group. In some instances, the patient may have evidence of a stroke (e.g., weakness of a limb), while in others the seizure may be the first and only sign of a stroke.

Other causes of seizures in the elderly include brain tumors, head trauma, and Alzheimer's disease. In particular, patients with Alzheimer's disease have a greater chance for seizures as the disorder progresses. Identification of the cause of new-onset seizures in the elderly is important because it can help to focus treatment. For example, if the seizures is found to be the first indication of an unrecognized disorder such as small tumor, treatment may be life-saving. Unfortunately, even using the newer methods of diagnosis, in as many as 30% to 40% of older patients, new-onset seizures do not have an apparent cause.

Diagnostic Testing

Once an unprovoked seizure has been diagnosed in a given patient, the physician must look for a cause. As with children and adults, we rely on imaging and the electroencephalogram (EEG) to find the source of the seizures. MRI is the best test to look for a lesion in the brain. As described in Chapter 2 , an MRI will find tumors, scar tissue, malformations, and evidence of strokes. The EEG can confirm the diagnosis of seizures by showing areas of the brain that are irritable.

Treatment

New-onset seizures in the elderly have a high chance of recurring because they typically arise from a *lesion* (abnormality) in the brain. Thus, the risk is high for seizures recurring even after a single unprovoked seizure in an elderly patient. Because of that, it is common to begin treatment after the first seizure in an elderly patient. The high risk for recurrence is a key difference of new seizures in the elderly as opposed to seizures in younger adults or children. However, even if the risk is high, the chances for adequate control are very good with current drugs.

Selecting an AED for an elderly patient is even more important than for a child since life-long treatment may be needed. Physician selection of an initial drug for an elderly patient must take into consideration how well the patient will tolerate the drug and its potential side effects, as well as how effective the drug will be at stopping seizures. In studies of patients with new-onset epileptic seizures, those seizures that are readily controlled are often controlled with relatively modest dosages.

Because most new seizures in the elderly are typically partial seizures with or without secondary generalization, almost all commonly used AEDs, both first and second generation, work well for partial seizures (see Chapters 4 and 5). A recent important study (VA trial 428) evaluated AED treatment of new-onset seizures in the elderly. This trial assessed how well the drugs worked and how well they were tolerated by the patient. The three drugs studied were gabapentin (Neurontin), lamotrigine (Lamictal), and carbamazepine (Tegretol). Carbamazepine, an older drug, is the most commonly used AED worldwide for the treatment of partial seizures. Gabapentin and lamotrigine are new-generation AEDs with good safety records. The trial showed no significant difference in how well each drug controlled seizures. Carbamazepine, however, was associated with significantly more *dropouts* (people stopping the medication) due to side effects (27%) compared with gabapentin (17%) or lamotrigine (10%). These results suggest that the newer drugs should be considered in initial treatment of the elderly because they are better tolerated.

An obvious question that arises is whether any of the newer AEDs are better than older AEDs for decreasing or stopping seizures. Nine new oral AEDs have been introduced in the United States since 1993. Unfortunately, only very few studies have compared the new AEDs with the older AEDs. In each of these studies, no significant differences have been shown on how effective the drugs are at treating seizures. Therefore, at present, the decision regarding AED selection should focus on safety and side effects.

Initial treatment should use only one drug (*monotherapy*). The American Academy of Neurology and the American Epilepsy Society, two very important medical societies in the United States, have issued guidelines for the treatment of new-onset and difficult epilepsy using newer AEDs. The guidelines support the use of gabapentin (Neurontin), lamotrigine (Lamictal), and topiramate (Topamax) as starting treatment for partial or mixed seizures, even though formal U.S. Food and Drug Administration (FDA) approval does not exist yet.

Elderly patients are more sensitive to adverse side effects in general, and these effects may occur at lower drug doses. Side effects such as unsteadiness, tremor, and sleepiness are common but often difficult to pinpoint in elderly patients with memory problems. Elderly patients typically are taking other medications for health problems other than seizures. One study found that elderly patients treated with AEDs were also taking an average of five other medications. These *co-medications* increase the risk for drug interactions with AEDs, which may create new health problems.

Use of Antiepileptic Drugs in the Elderly

For details on AEDs, see Chapters 4 and 5. Here we only highlight the most important points regarding AEDs and their use in the elderly.

Phenobarbital and Primidone (Mysoline)

Phenobarbital and primidone (which is converted to phenobarbital by the liver) are sedatives. In general, these are not a good choice as initial treatment for elderly patients.

Phenytoin (Dilantin)

Phenytoin (Dilantin) is the most widely prescribed AED in the United States. Phenytoin has several potentially severe disadvantages for the elderly, including an increased risk for *osteoporosis* (brittle bones). In addition, the metabolism of phenytoin is very peculiar; it's extremely difficult to find the proper effective dose, and it's very easy to overdose. Since phenytoin is cleared by the liver, many other drugs will affect and can be affected by its use. These factors have made many physicians stop prescribing phenytoin (Dilantin) for the elderly.

Carbamazepine (Tegretol)

Worldwide, carbamazepine is the most commonly used AED to treat partial seizures. Carbamazepine (Tegretol) does not pose the same problems as phenytoin, but it is metabolized by the liver and thus makes potential drug interactions a significant problem. For example, fluoxetine (Prozac) and even grapefruit juice can significantly increase carbamazepine blood levels to toxic levels. Lower sodium concentrations in blood (a condition known as *hyponatremia*) can be produced by carbamazepine, a side effect that is more common in the elderly. Sedation and osteoporosis are also important side effects that are of concern in the elderly.

Valproic Acid (Valproate, Depakote)

Valproate is commonly used in Europe as an AED. Although rare, liver toxicity can occur. *Tremor* of the hands is a common side effect, and since many elderly patients may already have tremor, it can make it worse. Valproate has less interactions with other drugs and does not induce osteoporosis and for that reason, it can be a good choice for some patients.

Gabapentin (Neurontin)

Gabapentin is one of the newer AEDs and has potential advantages over some of the older drugs. First, it is extremely safe, has very few side effects, and needs very little monitoring, which makes this drug an attractive choice for the elderly patient. Although it is not a powerful drug, it can work fairly well for the older patient, since seizures in the elderly are easier to control than in younger patients. It is, however, sedative and that can be a problem for patients already compromised by memory problems. Gabapentin may occasionally cause swelling of the extremities or weight gain.

Levetiracetam (Keppra)

Levetiracetam is one of the newer AEDs. It presents no safety or serious side-effect issues, and has no interactions with and is not affected by other medications. It has an excellent cognitive profile and rarely causes toxicity. Levetiracetam may be associated with mild irritability and psychiatric side effects, but these are rare and uncommon in the elderly. Levetiracetam is also now available for intravenous injection, thus making it a good choice for those unable to drink or eat.

Lamotrigine (Lamictal)

Lamotrigine offers many of the same benefits of gabapentin and levetiracetam. It is well tolerated, has few side effects, and doesn't cause cognitive problems. Several studies showed that lamotrigine is better tolerated than carbamazepine in elderly patients with new-onset seizures. Lamotrigine is approved as a mood stabilizer, and since depression is a common problem in the elderly and in patients with epilepsy, it can have a major beneficial impact on quality of life. Although the most serious side effect is rash, if introduced slowly, the risk of rash is extremely small. Lamotrigine is not sedative and thus a very good choice for elderly patients with cognitive impairment.

Oxcarbazepine (Trileptal)

Oxcarbazepine works very similarly to carbamazepine but is better tolerated and has a much lower risk of causing bone marrow problems such as anemia and low white cell counts. Drug interactions also are fewer than with carbamazepine. The major concern with oxcarbazepine in the elderly is the increased risk for inducing low sodium levels (*hyponatremia*) in the blood. About 5% to 10% of people taking oxcarbazepine develop low sodium levels, and because many elderly patients take diuretics (which tend to reduce sodium levels), the risk is even higher. Because of this, oxcarbazepine should be used with caution in elderly patients.

Topiramate (Topamax) and Zonisamide (Zonegran)

Topiramate and zonisamide have more cognitive side effects than the other AEDs discussed and thus are not drugs normally prescribed for elderly patients. When it's necessary to try topiramate and zonisamide, these side effects can be reduced by starting very slow and using lower doses. Both drugs have few serious side effects but both can induce kidney stones. Therefore, they are not appropriate in patients with a history of previous kidney stones. Both these AEDs can induce weight loss, which could be either a problem or an advantage depending on the patient's weight. Zonisamide can be taken once a day, which is an advantage.

BRAIN TUMORS AND EPILEPSY

Seizures are a common and sometimes devastating complication of brain tumors, and meticulous attention to their diagnosis and treatment is critical. The frequency of seizures is common in patients with brain tumors and is related to tumor location and probably to tumor type. Brain tumors are divided between *primary*, which originate in the brain, and *secondary*, which start elsewhere in the body and migrate to the brain (*metastasis*). Most brain tumors are either gliomas (which are *malignant*, or cancerous) or meningiomas (which are *benign*, or noncancerous). For primary brain tumors, epilepsy occurs in more than 80% of patients with low-grade gliomas, in 30% to 60% of patients with higher-grade gliomas (more malignant), and in as many as 40% of patients with meningiomas. Low grade and *cortical* (in close proximity to the cerebral cortex) tumor location are the main risk factors for epilepsy. Brain tumor patients who have epilepsy are significantly younger than older patients with tumors (without seizures) but it is unclear why this is the case.

As expected, most tumor-associated seizures are initially focal (originating from a specific location in the brain), although *generalization* (causing epileptic electrical discharges throughout the brain) may occur so quickly that the focal phase passes unnoticed. Seizure generalization is observed in one-half of the patients at the onset of the disease. Seizures may be the first sign of a brain tumor, although in most patients, other signs, such as headaches or dizziness, are the first signs of a brain tumor. If a patient is diagnosed as having a brain tumor, but does not have seizures, it's unlikely that seizures will develop later in the course of the illness. Because patients with brain tumor often have surgery or radiation treatments, the chance of developing seizures may differ from patient to patient.

Use of AEDs in Brain Tumor

Although the use of AEDs in patients with brain tumors is widespread, it is difficult to know if their use is necessary before seizures occur. Common practice is that, once a patient is diagnosed with a brain tumor, he is placed on an AED. The available evidence suggests, however, that *prophylactic* administration of anticonvulsant medications (medications given to prevent a problem, rather than to treat an existing problem) only reduces the risk of developing seizures by about 25%. On the other hand, the side effects associated with AEDs are fairly common and can be serious.

If a patient with a brain tumor develops seizures, then treatment with an AED is necessary. The choice of AED will depend on multiple factors including age, gender, and other drugs being taken. AEDs such as levetiracetam (Keppra) and gabapentin (Neurontin) are good first choices because they pose little risk of interacting with other medications. Unfortunately, despite AED treatment, many patients with brain tumors continue to have seizures, very often because of drug interactions with chemotherapy and steroid treatments that may change the amount of AED circulating in the blood. For this reason, careful monitoring of drug levels is often necessary.

BONE HEALTH AND EPILEPSY

Osteoporosis—a weakening of the bones—is another problem worthy of special comment. Although more commonly seen in women, both old and young, osteoporosis can affect men as well. *Estrogen*, a hormone produced in the bodies of both sexes, is responsible for good bone health. Because drugs that suppress estrogen are commonly used to treat breast cancer, osteoporosis is common in breast cancer survivors. And because postmenopausal women are no longer routinely prescribed estrogen replacement medications, older women are also at increased risk for osteoporosis.

Several older AEDs, such as carbamazepine, phenobarbital, phenytoin, and primidone, are most commonly associated with osteoporosis. These drugs increase the metabolism of vitamin D, which is a crucial vitamin that helps to deposit calcium in the bones and keep them strong.

The newer AEDs have little effect on vitamin D metabolism and therefore don't pose the same risk of osteoporosis.

Osteoporosis can lead to fractures—in particular, hip fractures, which are a serious medical problem in the elderly. Death from complications of hip fracture in the elderly can occur in about 20% of people. A recent study estimated that women taking phenytoin had a 30% increased risk for hip fractures over 5 years compared with women not taking this AED.

Osteoporosis cannot be detected unless bone density scans are done. Unfortunately, most patients receive a diagnosis of osteoporosis *after* a fracture has taken place. Avoiding AEDs that promote osteoporosis is recommended in the elderly, in postmenopausal women, and in patients who are immobile (because immobility increases the chance of osteoporosis). If these AEDs must be used, bone mineral density should be measured and monitored, and supplemental vitamin D and calcium should be prescribed. Some physicians also recommend vitamin D and calcium supplements for any patient who is taking medications to treat liver disorders.

FREQUENTLY ASKED QUESTIONS

Q What are common causes of seizures in elderly patients?

A Elderly patients have an increased risk for seizures and epilepsy. The most common cause of epilepsy in this group is stroke. Other causes include tumors, trauma and infections.

Q Which are the best antiepileptic drugs for an elderly individual?

A There is no simple answer that the question. Each patient should receive a particular drug depending on their condition, number of other drugs that is taking, and other variables. Certainly the trend is to use drugs that are not sedative and are easy to use while taking other medications.

Q Should a patient taking phenytoin (Dilantin) for many years be on Vitamin D and Calcium supplements?

A Although there are no strict guidelines on the use of Vit D and calcium for patients with epilepsy, the consensus among many specialists is that Vit D and Calcium may help reverse some of the effects of phenytoin on bone health and thus, it is recommended.

My Notes

10

LIVING WITH EPILEPSY

Addressing Common Concerns

Key Points

▶ Antiepileptic drugs side effects can change a person's overall quality of life.

▶ Epilepsy can cause you to have alterations in sleep.

▶ People with epilepsy are protected by the Americans with Disabilities Act of 1990.

▶ Seizures can interfere with a child's ability to learn at the same pace as other children his age.

▶ A healthy diet is essential for everyone, especially for people with epilepsy.

LIVING WITH EPILEPSY IS A CHALLENGE. Your work, activities, transportation, education, diet, memory, and even sleep are different from that of people without epilepsy. This chapter discusses these issues and provides patients with good resources to assist you in dealing with them. Whether you are newly diagnosed or have had epilepsy for years, this chapter will benefit both you and your family.

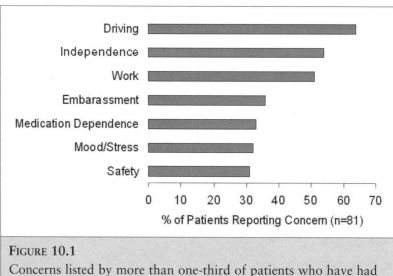

FIGURE 10.1
Concerns listed by more than one-third of patients who have had one or more seizures in the past 6 months.

Epilepsy may affect many aspects of a person's life. Although the challenge of living with epilepsy may solidify family ties or allow a more empathetic perspective toward others, most of the effects of epilepsy put limits on an individual's goals and aspirations. Over the past decade, researchers from around the world have attempted to identify the most important concerns of persons living with epilepsy. The most commonly identified areas of concern include transportation, personal independence, social embarrassment, safety, mood, and medication problems (Fig. 10.1). To help you talk about your own concerns with your physician, you may want to use the short form shown in Figure 10.2.

In addition to physicians, *advocates* are working through the legal system to improve the overall quality of life for people with epilepsy. The Americans with Disabilities Act of 1990 is an important piece of legislation that applies to people with epilepsy. This act aims to eliminate discrimination against the more than 43 million Americans with disabilities. It addresses employment, public transportation, housing, education, recreation, health services, and other issues. Persons with epilepsy are entitled to the rights protected under this act. Your disability gives you additional protection from discrimination. For example, if epilepsy prevents you from driving, this act allows you to access certain community resources, such as paratransit vehicles, to transport you when you are unable to drive. For more information on rights for disabled Americans, visit www.disabilityinfo.gov or www.disabilityresources.org.

EFA Concerns Index

Name _____ Date _____

Patient's ID# _____ Gender _____ Birth Date _____

Instructions: .

This questionnaire asks about your concerns of living with epilepsy. Please answer every question by circling the appropriate number (1, 2, 3, 4, or 5).

If you are unsure of an answer to a question, please give your best response.

You may write comments in the margin to explain your answer if needed.

1–13: For each of the PROBLEMS listed below, circle one number for how much they have concerned you during the past 4 weeks on a scale of 1 to 5, where 1 = Not concerned at all, and 5 = Extremely concerned.

		Not at all Concerned				Extremely Concerned
1.	your legal right or ability to drive	1	2	3	4	5
2.	fear of being injured during a seizure	1	2	3	4	5
3.	having to take seizure medications	1	2	3	4	5
4.	holding down a job	1	2	3	4	5
5.	getting the work or education you want	1	2	3	4	5
6.	not being able to do things alone	1	2	3	4	5
7.	having a seizure unexpectedly	1	2	3	4	5
8.	being treated unfairly by others	1	2	3	4	5
9.	being a burden or worry to your family	1	2	3	4	5
10.	medical costs of your epilepsy	1	2	3	4	5
11.	effects of your epilepsy on your family	1	2	3	4	5
12.	your future	1	2	3	4	5
13.	lack of other people's understanding of epilepsy	1	2	3	4	5

continues on next page

FIGURE 10.2
A "concerns form" to share with your physician.

14–20: During the past 4 weeks, have you...

	None of the time	Some of the time	A good bit of the time	Most of the time	All of the time
14. been worried about having another seizure?	1	2	3	4	5
15. had problems with medication side effects?	1	2	3	4	5
16. felt embarrassed about your seizures?	1	2	3	4	5
17. been unable to do things "for fun" that you wanted to do?	1	2	3	4	5
18. had problems thinking or remembering?	1	2	3	4	5
19. felt nervous, depressed, or "stressed out" because of your seizures?	1	2	3	4	5
20. had difficulty obtaining transportation?	1	2	3	4	5

Comments:

FIGURE 10.2
A "concerns form" to share with your physician.

MANAGING ANTIEPILEPTIC DRUG SIDE EFFECTS

Antiepileptic drugs (AEDs) are a necessary component of epilepsy treatment. For most people, seizures are decreased and may ultimately stop completely with these medications. These drugs, however, cause undesirable side effects for many people. Some side effects disappear after a few weeks of taking the drug while others persist. Depending on which drug you are taking, you could experience fatigue, weight gain, mood changes, memory changes, abnormal hair growth, or other adverse effects. Some drug side effects are unavoidable. However, in other cases, your doctor can alleviate side effects by changing the medications you take. You should always consult your doctor regarding other medications if your side effects are affecting your lifestyle in ways that are unacceptable to you. If your body reacts poorly to one drug, other options may be open to you.

The way these drugs interact with your body may be different from the way they behave in another person. You are an individual and should be treated as such.

Experiencing side effects from AEDs generally occurs when a new drug is started or with increasing dosage. You should be aware of the side effects of the particular drug that you are taking. Please refer to Chapter 3 and 4 for a complete list. Although side effects may decrease with time, there are several methods to help you handle them in your daily life.

Fatigue

▶ Try establishing a normal sleep pattern. Keep the time you go to sleep and the time you wake up the same every day (including weekends).

▶ Moderate amounts of exercise may help your body to feel less stressed and less tired.

▶ Make sure you do not let the fatigue keep you from eating healthy foods. Your diet can help lessen fatigue. Try keeping ready-to-eat or easy-to-cook foods handy so that you can eat well even when you do not have the energy to prepare a meal.

Skin Changes (Rash or Sun Sensitivity)

▶ Avoid extra-hot showers and baths since hot water may irritate your skin further.

▶ Avoid excessive sun exposure and always wear sunscreen and protective clothing.

Headache

▶ To relieve a headache:
  ▷ Try resting in a quiet place with minimal light and noise.
    Place a cold washcloth over your forehead and eyes.

▶ To avoid a headache:
  ▷ Observe possible triggers of your headaches and attempt to avoid them. For example, bright lights, certain foods, and caffeine can trigger a headache.

Hair Loss

▶ Try to avoid or limit the use of certain hair care practices such as dyeing, straightening, or braiding your hair.

▶ Attempt to decrease your amount of stress because this can worsen hair loss.

Upset Stomach

▶ Place crackers by your bedside and eat a few when you wake up in the morning. Sit in your bed for a few minutes after you eat them.

▶ Try certain stomach-soothing teas, such as ginger, chamomile, or peppermint.

▶ Slowly sip a carbonated beverage, such as ginger ale or Sprite.

▶ Avoid spicy, strong smelling, and greasy foods.

Weight Changes

▶ Establish a regular exercise routine of at least 30 minutes of activity three times a week.
▶ Avoid eating more food than you usually consume. Try to eat healthy foods on a regular basis.

Memory Difficulties

▶ Try using memory aids:
  ▷ Use sticky notes to remind yourself of appointments or things to do. Place the notes where you will see them, such as on the front door or refrigerator.
  ▷ Keep an appointment book and to-do list to help keep track of your schedule for the day.
  ▷ Use pill boxes with the days of the week to help you remember your daily medications. Use a separate box for morning, afternoon, and night doses. Place the meds in a place where you will see them and remember to take them. For example, place your morning and night meds by your toothbrush so that you will take them when you perform other routine hygiene tasks.
  ▷ Use a tape recorder to tell yourself about appointments or things you have to do. Most cellular phones have an option to use your voice to record a memo. When you need to remember some information, you can leave yourself a message on your cell phone. Check your phone daily to listen to your reminders.
  ▷ Ask a family member or co-worker to remind you of things to do or appointments you must keep.
▶ Remembering names:
  ▷ Try repeating the person's name to yourself multiple times when you meet them.
  ▷ Try associating the person's name with an image or object that will help you remember it.
▶ Forgetting where you placed objects:
  ▷ Try to keep things you commonly use in the same place all the time.
  ▷ When you put an object in a new place, take the time to focus on where you put it, so it will be easier to recall its location when you need the item again.

AED side effects change a person's overall quality of life. The ultimate goal of your physician is to stop your seizures. In this process, however, the side effects of the drugs you are prescribed are often overlooked. Of course, you want your seizures stopped too, but living with intolerable drug side effects is not acceptable. This crucial difference in ideas of what constitutes successful treatment can be a problem, so it is important to be an advocate for yourself. When you visit with your doctor, make sure that you have a list of the side effects that you are experiencing. The Adverse Events Profile table in Figure 10.3 will help you to do this. Fill out this table for each drug you are taking. For further information on AED side effects visit www.epilepsy.com/epilepsy/medicine_sideeffects.html or www.epilepsynse.org.uk/pages/info/leaflets/drug.cfm.

DRIVING LAWS

Imagine having a sales job that requires travel throughout the city to negotiate deals on a daily basis. How would you work if you were unable to drive? This is a question facing almost a million people with epilepsy in the United States on a daily basis. In a country where most cities lack a good public transportation system, driving a car is a necessity of daily life. Being able to drive gives a person both independence and the ability to be self-sufficient. Both of these characteristics are highly valued in our society. Adults with epilepsy and their family members acknowledge that the most difficult and debilitating aspect of having uncontrolled seizures is the inability to drive.

Driving regulations for people with seizures vary from state to state. Generally, you can expect to be prohibited from driving for up to 12 months following a seizure. This is a necessary mandate by the state to keep both you and other people on the roads safe. Accidents can occur if a person has a seizure while driving a car. A recent study reviewing fatal car crashes from 1995 to 1997 revealed that 0.2% (86) of the 44,027 deaths involved drivers with epilepsy. Despite this seemingly small fraction of epilepsy-associated automobile fatalities, it is still important to restrict people with active seizures from driving. In most states, it is not required for your physician to report that you have had a seizure. Therefore, it is your responsibility to know your seizure record and follow the laws in your state regarding driving. To find out what your state's laws are regarding driving restrictions after a seizure, visit www.epilepsy.com/epilepsy/rights_driving.

Although alternative modes of transportation are available, locating and utilizing these resources can be frustrating. According to the Americans with Disabilities Act of 1990, you are eligible for services such as paratransit systems. These are vehicles that will pick you up and transport you to your required destination for a minimal cost. This service is available in most cities that lack easily accessible public transportation. The United States lacks a central system for dealing with the issue of transportation for people with disabilities. However, the following list of resources may help you to locate available methods of transportation in your area.

▶ www.ctaa.org/ntrc/accessibility/weblinks.asp. This web site offers links to available transportation for people with disabilities. National as well as state programs are listed.

▶ www.paratransit.net. This web site offers information for paratransit systems in Oregon, California, Alaska, and Washington. Although this will not be helpful to everyone, you can use an Internet search engine to locate a paratransit system in your area.

Adverse Events Profile

During the past 4 weeks, have you had any of the problems or side-effects listed below?

For each item, if it has always or often been a problem, circle 4; if it has sometimes been a problem, circle 3; and so on. Please be sure to answer every item.

	Always or often a problem	Sometimes a problem	Rarely a problem	Never a problem
Unsteadiness	4	3	2	1
Tiredness	4	3	2	1
Restlessness	4	3	2	1
Feelings of aggression	4	3	2	1
Nervousness and/or agitation	4	3	2	1
Headache	4	3	2	1
Hair loss	4	3	2	1
Problems with skin, e.g. acne, rash	4	3	2	1
Double or blurred vision	4	3	2	1
Upset stomach	4	3	2	1
Difficulty in concentrating	4	3	2	1
Trouble with mouth or gums	4	3	2	1
Shaky hands	4	3	2	1
Weight gain	4	3	2	1
Dizziness	4	3	2	1
Sleepiness	4	3	2	1
Depression	4	3	2	1
Memory problems	4	3	2	1
Disturbed sleep	4	3	2	1

FIGURE 10.3
Adverse events profile.

▶   www.publictransportation.org/systems. This site links you to community public transportation in each state.

▶   www.tlpa.org/findaride/index.cfm. This is the web site of the Taxicab, Limousine & Paratransit Association (TLPA). It allows you to select both domestic and international locations, and it will give you the transportation options for that area.

▶   http://projectaction.easterseals.com/cgi-bin/traveler_search.cgi. This is a database of accessible community transportation for all 50 states and most major cities within each state. The database has all available companies' information in each state.

ALCOHOL USE

The recreational use of alcohol is common in almost every society. It is present at meals, work functions, and most social gatherings. While having epilepsy should not restrict you from drinking alcohol, your intake should be limited. There are no clear guidelines established regarding the amount of alcohol acceptable for persons with epilepsy. It appears that one drink, especially with a large meal, is well tolerated by most people. The concern most physicians hold is that alcohol can potentially increase your chance of having a seizure. It can also interact with your antiepileptic medicines.

A statement from the National Institute on Alcohol Abuse and Alcoholism points out that many medications interact with alcohol, which can lead to injury, illness, or even death. It notes that for some AEDs specifically, a definite interaction is known. For instance, acute alcohol consumption increases the risk of reaching toxic blood levels of phenytoin (Dilantin), which can cause an increase in drug side effects. With long-term use of both alcohol and Dilantin, blood levels of the drug decrease, necessitating higher doses of the medication to achieve the desired seizure control. Having epilepsy does not mean you cannot have alcohol, but be sure to discuss the topic with your physician.

SLEEP AND SEIZURES

Epilepsy can cause you to have alterations in sleep. You may feel tired all the time and find yourself needing extra naps just to function during the day. You may also find that, despite spending an adequate amount of time in bed at night, you do not feel rested in the morning. These sleep complaints are common and are caused by a number of different factors. Epilepsy itself can cause changes in your natural sleep pattern. Researchers believe that an inadequate amount of sleep, poor sleep hygiene, sleep disorders, AEDs, and interruptions in natural sleep patterns can all cause problems.

Fatigue is a common difficulty for people with epilepsy. It is not normal to experience excessive fatigue. This tiredness interferes with your ability to interact with your surroundings and with other people. If you find that you require frequent naps or an increase in the amount of hours you spend in bed at night, you should notify your physician. This tiredness could be a side effect of one of your drugs. If this is the case, it may be possible to adjust your dose or change your medicine. However, fatigue can also be the result of an underlying sleep disorder. Many people with epilepsy also suffer from an underlying sleep disorder such as obstructive *sleep apnea* or restless leg syndrome. Both of these disorders can be diag-

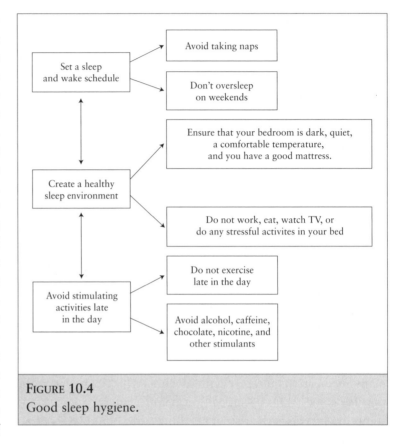

FIGURE 10.4
Good sleep hygiene.

nosed with a sleep study and are treatable conditions. Once treated, your overall quality of sleep should improve, and your daytime fatigue should decrease significantly.

Poor sleep hygiene is common among many individuals, but as a person with epilepsy, it can be detrimental to your health. Sleep disturbances may cause seizures to occur despite adequate medication. It is essential that you learn good sleep habits. Figure 10.4 details good sleep hygiene.

EMPLOYMENT AND DISCLOSURE OF EPILEPSY

The unemployment rate for people with epilepsy is higher than that of the general population. In a society that values one's ability to work, this fact is particularly distressing to persons with epilepsy. Being able to hold a successful job can give a person a sense of self worth. Quality-of-life scores are diminished in many people with epilepsy who do not have a job. The reason for this decreased rate of employment is not clear. However, it is likely that someone with seizures may have difficulty working if they require a significant amount of medicine, or if their seizures are not controlled. Another reason may be that it is difficult for a person with epilepsy to overcome the stigma that can be associated with their disease. Employers and co-workers may not be educated regarding the disease and may therefore have negative attitudes about your ability to work effectively. These reasons may cause you to decide against disclosing your illness in the workplace.

The decision to discuss your illness with your employer and co-workers is challenging. Many people with epilepsy are concerned that they will be discriminated against when applying for a new job or promotion based on their illness. People with epilepsy are protected by the Americans with Disabilities Act of 1990. Under the Act, it is unlawful for an employer to discriminate against a qualified applicant or employee with a disability. As an applicant you must, however, meet the employer's qualifications for the job, including education, training, experience, and skills. For more information regarding the ADA and employment visitwww.eeoc.gov/facts/jobapplicant.html.

Web sites also are available to help you with your decision to disclose your illness:

▶   www.onestops.info/print.php?article_id=107. Offers rules for good disclosure of a nonapparent or hidden disability.
▶   www.epilepsyfoundation.org/epilepsyusa/disclosure.cfm. Discusses issues of disclosure and attitudes regarding epilepsy in the workplace.
▶   www.epilepsyinstitute.org/faq/main.htm. Helps you construct multiple scenarios to assist you in disclosing your illness.

The chart in Figure 10.5, created by the Epilepsy Foundation, can further assist you in your decision.

EXERCISE

The overall level of activity and fitness in people with epilepsy is decreased in comparison to the general population. Studies show that people with epilepsy participate in fewer sports, have decreased muscle and aerobic strength, and have a higher body mass index compared with people without epilepsy. Another study found that people with at least one seizure a month were half as active as the average population. These statistics are not ideal for a group that already has significant health issues.

The importance of exercise in everyday life cannot be stressed enough. Exercise improves the body's ability to fight disease, overcome fatigue, and maintain a healthy body weight. It can also improve the quality of sleep a person achieves each night. Also, because people with epilepsy have increased bone fragility (*osteoporosis*), exercise, especially resistance training, can improve your bone health. It can also improve your overall health and help you to fight your disease and improve your quality of life.

Time of Disclosure	Advantages	Disadvantages	Issues
On a job application. (If the employer is covered by the ADA or Rehabilitation Act the request for information is voluntary. If covered by a state law, such questions may be legal.)	Honesty/peace of mind.	Might disqualify you with no opportunity to present yourself and your qualifications. Potential for discrimination.	Do you know what legal protections are in place regarding information requested on a job application? Need to do some basic research before applying for some jobs. Early disclosure may avoid problems once you are hired.
During an interview.	Opportunity to respond briefly and positively in person to specific issues. Can raise issue of accommodations you need or the fact that your epilepsy won't interfere with your job.	Puts responsibility on you to handle epilepsy issues clearly. Too much talk on the issue may indicate possible problem. Not being evaluated on your abilities.	How comfortable are you with discussing your epilepsy? These are very difficult questions but ones that you can prepare to answer.
After the interview. (When a job is offered but before you begin work.)	If the disclosure changes the hiring decision and you are sure of your ability, then you may take legal action for discrimination.	Might lead to distrust.	Need to evaluate your seizure condition in light of your job duties. Need to explain how epilepsy will not interfere with ability to perform job.

FIGURE 10.5
Disclosing epilepsy to your employer.

Time of Disclosure	Advantages	Disadvantages	Issues
After you start work.	Opportunity to prove yourself on job before disclosure. Allows you to respond to epilepsy questions with peers at work. If disclosure affects employment status and the condition doesn't affect ability to perform job or job safety, you may be protected by law.	Nervousness or fear of having a seizure on the job. Possible employer accusation of falsifying your application. Could change interaction with peers.	The longer you put off disclosing the harder it becomes. It may be difficult to identify whom to tell.
After a seizure on the job.	Opportunity to prove yourself on the job before disclosure. If disclosure affects employment status and the condition doesn't affect ability to perform job or job safety, you may be protected by law.	Possible employer accusation for falsifying your application. Possibility that your co-workers will not know how to react to your seizure.	You should be prepared to answer questions from your employer and co-workers about epilepsy and why you didn't tell them.
Never.	Employer can't respond to your epilepsy unless you have a seizure.	Nervousness or fear of having a seizure on the job.	If you haven't had a seizure for a long time (like over 1 to 2 years) the issue of disclosure becomes less critical.

This page is from the Epilepsy Foundation© web site and can be viewed at www.epilepsyfoundation.org/programs/disclosure.cfm

FIGURE 10.5
Disclosing epilepsy to your employer.

It is common for someone with epilepsy to be advised to refrain from strenuous activity because it may provoke a seizure. You can, however, engage in physical activities that will improve your health without affecting your seizure rate. To avoid exercise-induced seizure triggers, be sure to follow these instructions:

▶ Always drink plenty of water to keep your body hydrated.
▶ If you feel that you are overexerting yourself, stop the activity and rest.
▶ Make sure that you rest on several days of the week.
▶ Maintain a healthy diet.
▶ Ensure that you are getting adequate sleep and are not fatigued.

Prior to starting a new exercise regimen, consult your doctor. Your exercise regimen should include the three main types of exercise: aerobic, resistance training, and stretching. You should attempt to do at least 30 minutes of aerobic exercise three times a week. This could include walking, jogging, or using a stair-climbing machine. You should attempt to do 20 to 30 minutes of resistance training twice a week. This includes using weight machines or resistance bands. The third element of exercise—stretching—should be done at the end of every workout session. Make sure to include all of your major muscle groups when you stretch. Be sure to start exercising at a level that is comfortable for you. You can increase the time and frequency of your workout as your body adjusts. The benefits to your health from exercising far outweigh the potential risks, but try to avoid the risky exercises listed here:

▶ Motor sports
▶ Horseback riding
▶ Gymnastics
▶ Ice activities, such as skating or hockey
▶ Skiing
▶ Solo water sports, such as sailing or wind surfing
▶ Water activities, such as swimming, alone

For information on low-, moderate-, and high-risk sports, and on those sports that require a helmet, visit www.epilepsy.ca/eng/content/teens.html.

SAFETY

It may be frustrating to you, as a person with epilepsy, that everyone seems overly concerned about your safety. Your family and friends may take extra precautions to ensure that you avoid activities that could be seizure triggers. They are also concerned that you may experience an epilepsy-related injury. Studies show that it is common for a person to be injured during a seizure. These injuries include burns, dental trauma, and bone fractures. There is reason for concern, but there are some things that you can do to decrease your risk of injury:

Safety 101 Checklist

▶ Keep all bathroom and bedroom doors unlocked.
▶ Turn down the hot water temperature in your house.
▶ Take showers, *not* baths.
▶ Avoid heights and stay off ladders.
▶ Don't carry hot pots or pans from the oven or stove—bring your plate to the stove.
▶ Use microwave cooking as much as possible.
▶ Place handles to pots and saucepans toward the center of the stove.
▶ Avoid fireplaces or hot radiators.
▶ Stay clear of furniture with sharp edges.

DIET

A healthy diet is essential to everyone, especially for people with epilepsy. It is common to experience weight gain with some of your medicines. By watching what you eat, you will be able to avoid this effect. The U.S. Department of Agriculture published a new food pyramid recently that puts an emphasis on whole grains, vegetables, and fruits. It allows for sparing amounts of fats and meats. Refer to the nutrition guide in Figure 10.6 to help you develop a healthy diet.

Several foods and food additives should be avoided by people with epilepsy. Certain foods, such as grapefruit juice, can interact with specific AEDs. Check with your doctor to see if any of these restrictions apply to you. It is a common misconception that some food additives can cause seizures. One example is aspartame, an artificial sweetener in many diet drinks. Multiple studies with animals and humans have determined that there is no evidence that this is true. It is safe to use aspartame. To date, no known foods or food additives trigger seizures in large numbers of people with epilepsy.

EDUCATION ISSUES FOR CHILDREN

Seizures can interfere with a child's ability to learn at the same pace as other children his age. Children can feel isolated and different from their peers as a result. The seizures can make them miss parts of class, experience extreme fatigue, and have trouble with memory. Government programs and agencies are available to assist your child in receiving the education he deserves.

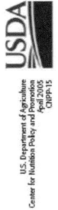

GRAINS
Make half your grains whole

Eat at least 3 oz. of whole-grain cereals, breads, crackers, rice, or pasta every day

1 oz. is about 1 slice of bread, about 1 cup of breakfast cereal, or ½ cup of cooked rice, cereal, or pasta

VEGETABLES
Vary your veggies

Eat more dark-green veggies like broccoli, spinach, and other dark leafy greens

Eat more orange vegetables like carrots and sweetpotatoes

Eat more dry beans and peas like pinto beans, kidney beans, and lentils

FRUITS
Focus on fruits

Eat a variety of fruit

Choose fresh, frozen, canned, or dried fruit

Go easy on fruit juices

MILK
Get your calcium-rich foods

Go low-fat or fat-free when you choose milk, yogurt, and other milk products

If you don't or can't consume milk, choose lactose-free products or other calcium sources such as fortified foods and beverages

MEAT & BEANS
Go lean with protein

Choose low-fat or lean meats and poultry

Bake it, broil it, or grill it

Vary your protein routine – choose more fish, beans, peas, nuts, and seeds

For a 2,000-calorie diet, you need the amounts below from each food group. To find the amounts that are right for you, go to MyPyramid.gov.

| Eat 6 oz. every day | Eat 2½ cups every day | Eat 2 cups every day | Get 3 cups every day; for kids aged 2 to 8, it's 2 | Eat 5½ oz. every day |

Find your balance between food and physical activity
- Be sure to stay within your daily calorie needs.
- Be physically active for at least 30 minutes most days of the week.
- About 60 minutes a day of physical activity may be needed to prevent weight gain.
- For sustaining weight loss, at least 60 to 90 minutes a day of physical activity may be required.
- Children and teenagers should be physically active for 60 minutes every day, or most days.

Know the limits on fats, sugars, and salt (sodium)
- Make most of your fat sources from fish, nuts, and vegetable oils.
- Limit solid fats like butter, stick margarine, shortening, and lard, as well as foods that contain these.
- Check the Nutrition Facts label to keep saturated fats, trans fats, and sodium low.
- Choose food and beverages low in added sugars. Added sugars contribute calories with few, if any, nutrients.

MyPyramid.gov
STEPS TO A HEALTHIER YOU

USDA

U.S. Department of Agriculture
Center for Nutrition Policy and Promotion
April 2005
CNPP-15

USDA is an equal opportunity provider and employer.

FIGURE 10.6
A healthy-eating guide.

Students with epilepsy are eligible for special education and related services under the Individuals with Disabilities Education Act (IDEA). This act requires public schools to provide an education in the least restrictive environment that meets each individual child's needs. IDEA requires public school systems to develop appropriate Individualized Education Programs (IEPs) for each child. The specific special education and related services outlined in each IEP reflect the individual needs of each student.

For more information on programs regarding education visit:

▶ www.nichcy.org. The web site for the National Dissemination Center for Children with Disabilities.
▶ www.pacer.org. The web site for the Parent Advocacy Coalition for Educational Rights.
▶ www.ideapractices.org. The web site for the Council of Exceptional Children. This council advocates as the voice and vision of special education.

FREQUENTLY ASKED QUESTIONS

Q How long do I have to be seizure-free to be able to drive?

A The time restriction varies from state to state. In most states, it is 6 months, but it can be up to 1 year. Please ask your doctor about your particular situation and the state law.

Q Can I still drink alcohol?

A Alcohol is acceptable to drink in moderation. For example, one glass of wine or one beer with a meal should not affect your medicine. However, each patient is different and you should discuss with your doctor. Alcohol can interfere with some AED's and can also affect the metabolism of your liver.

Q Do I have to live with the side effects of my AEDs, such as extreme fatigue?

A No! Talk to your doctor if you are experiencing side effects that you cannot tolerate. Other drugs are available. Side effects are individual and every patient is different on how they react to medications. It is important that you tell your doctor any problems you may have with the medications.

Q Do I have to tell my boss that I have epilepsy?

A You are not legally required to tell your employer about your condition. It is your decision to determine if this is necessary.

Q Will my seizures cause permanent or progressive brain damage that will affect things like my speech?

A No. In most types of epilepsy, recurrent seizures will not cause progressive trouble with speech or motor function. It depends on many factors, location of seizures, medications, cause of your seizures, etc. Some patients do experience changes while the majority do not.

My Notes

_____

_____

_____

_____

_____

_____

_____

_____

_____

_____

11

Cognitive and Psychiatric Aspects

Recognition and Treatment

Key Points

▶ In epilepsy, many things can potentially produce adverse effects on cognitive abilities.

▶ The frequency, duration, and severity of seizures may affect cognition in several ways.

▶ Several recent studies in humans provide evidence that exposure to valproate during pregnancy poses a special risk for cognition.

▶ Attention deficit disorders (ADDs) are the most frequent psychiatric disorder identified in children with epilepsy, although they occur in adults as well.

COGNITION IN EPILEPSY

COGNITION REFERS TO ABILITIES such as intelligence, attention, memory, language, thinking speed, and ability to plan and problem solve. A recent survey in Europe by the International Bureau for Epilepsy found that 44% of patients with epilepsy complained of difficulty learning, 45% of slowed thinking, 59% of sedation, and 63% felt that their antiepileptic drugs (AEDs) prevented them from achieving activities or goals. A survey in the United States over a decade ago found similar results. Thus, the cognitive side effects of AEDs are clearly a problem. Most people with epilepsy have normal intelligence, and some even have superior intelligence. However, epilepsy is more common and more likely to be difficult to control in patients with mental retardation. In the general population, many things contribute to a person's cognitive abilities, such as genetic and environmental factors. In epilepsy, many things can potentially produce adverse effects on cognitive abilities. Table 11.1 lists factors that may affect cognition.

The cause of seizures may be one of the strongest factors influencing cognitive abilities. For example, if the seizures are due to progressive brain degeneration, patients will usually develop *dementia*. If the seizures are caused by brain injury (*trauma*), stroke, or tumor, the patient may have specific cognitive deficits. In contrast, if the cause of seizures is *idiopathic* (unknown),

---

TABLE 11.1

Factors That May Affect Cognition in People with Epilepsy

Underlying cause of seizures

Brain lesions acquired prior to onset of seizures

Type of seizures

Age at onset of epilepsy

Seizure frequency, duration, and severity

Impairments during and after seizures

Adverse effects of epileptic discharges between seizures

Brain damage from multiple seizures

Psychosocial factors resulting from epilepsy

Hereditary factors

Side effects of treatments for epilepsy such as surgery or AEDs

---

patients are more likely to have normal intelligence. Cognitive abilities have also been related to seizure type. For example, patients with *juvenile myoclonic epilepsy* usually have normal intelligence, but children with *infantile spasms* frequently have poor cognitive abilities. Overall, patients are more likely to have cognitive impairment if the first seizures occur at an earlier age.

The frequency, duration, and severity of seizures may affect cognition in several ways. During seizures, patients may lose consciousness or experience confusion. Following a seizure (the *postictal state*), a patient may be very confused or have problems with memory. This effect may last to some degree for minutes, hours, or even days. For example, patients who have had recent *temporal lobe seizures* may have increased problems with memory in the period following a seizure even after their confusion has resolved.

In a person with epilepsy, the abnormal electrical discharges in the brain that occur between seizures (during the interictal state) also may impair cognition, although the exact amount of impairment from these interictal discharges is uncertain. Nevertheless, it is clear that in some patients such discharges may cause very brief, passing reductions in cognitive performance. For example, children are more likely to make errors on a video game during brief runs of interictal discharges. Patients with *focal epilepsy* (seizure begin at one place in the brain) may have chronic dysfunction of the brain in that region. Further, the dysfunction may extend beyond the area of actual seizure onset. For example, *positron emission tomography* or PET scans can show reduced brain activity between seizures not only in the region of seizure onset (the *focal* region) but also extending to surrounding brain regions. This reduced activity can be reversed if the seizures are stopped. However, repetitive or prolonged seizures may permanently damage the brain.

Hereditary factors can strongly influence intelligence. The IQ (*intelligence quotient*) of a child's mother is the single most important factor in predicting that child's IQ. Other factors, such as the father's IQ, living conditions (*socioeconomic status*), and brain injuries also influence a child's IQ.

Psychosocial factors may affect cognition. For example, poor socioeconomic status during childhood can adversely affect cognitive development. Finally, therapies for epilepsy, such as surgery or AEDs, also may affect cognition. These will be discussed next.

Epilepsy Surgery

In people with epilepsy whose seizures are refractory to AEDs, epilepsy surgery may offer the best hope of freedom from seizures if the onset of seizures can be localized and the damaged area removed without producing new problems. The risk of postoperative cognitive problems depends on the function of the area of the brain that is to be removed (*resected*). For example, if the seizure focus involves language areas of the brain, removal could lead to forms of *aphasia*, such as difficulties with spontaneous speech, understanding words, naming, or reading. Even in this situation, aphasic problems may be reduced by mapping the brain to tailor the resection to avoid critical language areas or by performing a special type of surgical procedure known as *multiple subpial tran-*

sections. Fortunately, epilepsy surgery does not usually lead to general cognitive decline because the tissue removed at the focus frequently does not function well. Surgery may even result in improved cognition because of the reduction in seizures and need for AEDs.

The most common type of epilepsy surgery is *anterior temporal lobectomy.* The anterior medial temporal lobe has the lowest seizure threshold in the brain and is the most common site for the onset of focal epilepsy. Surgeons are very experienced in treating that area of the brain. However, anterior temporal lobectomy can result in postoperative cognitive problems. The medial temporal lobes are critical for forming new memories. If both temporal lobes are damaged, then the patient will become *amnestic* (unable to remember events on a day to day basis). As long as one temporal lobe remains functional, the patient will not become amnestic, although they might experience some decline in memory. The best candidates for anterior temporal lobectomy have seizures arising from a nonfunctional medial temporal lobe, with the temporal lobe on the opposite side of the brain functioning well. Therefore, the preoperative evaluation must determine if and how much of the temporal lobe to be removed contributes to memory and if the remaining temporal lobe can support memory.

Luckily, the risks are largely predictable. The occurrence of severe amnesia is extremely rare, and most patients undergoing temporal lobectomy will not suffer significant declines. A major concern in the preoperative evaluation is predicting even a partial decline in memory, especially *verbal memory* (the ability to remember words and names). The risks are greater if the patient's epilepsy started at an older age (not as an infant), or if hippocampal scarring and atrophy are not present. The risk of significant problems is higher if the language-dominant temporal lobe (usually the left side) is involved.

Preoperative assessments done by your doctors will be used to predict what sort of memory problems may occur following surgery. These assessments may include the *Wada test*, PET scans, or *functional MRI* (magnetic resonance imaging) scans. The Wada test is also called the *intracarotid amobarbital test.* To perform the Wada test, the physician threads a very small tube (a *catheter*) up from the big arteries in the leg to the carotid arteries in the neck. A short-acting anesthetic agent such as amobarbital is injected. This basically puts one side of the brain to sleep for a few minutes so that language and memory function can be assessed. The point is to determine which side of the brain controls language and how much each side contributes to memory. New *noninvasive techniques* such as functional MRI may soon replace the *invasive* Wada test. The PET scan measures the *metabolism* (activity) of the brain. The finding of *hypometabolism* (low activity) in one medial temporal lobe is consistent with a seizure focus and reduced function on that side.

Vagal Nerve Stimulation

Vagal nerve stimulation (VNS) can reduce seizures, although patients rarely become seizure free. VNS does not appear to produce any adverse cognitive effects. Refer to Chapter 5 for more information.

Antiepileptic Drugs

AEDs control seizures by reducing nerve cell irritability, but they can also affect cognition by suppressing nerve cell excitability. In general, the cognitive side effects of AEDs are mild, especially when only one AED is prescribed (monotherapy). The main cognitive side effects of AEDs include slowing of motor and cognitive speed, reduced attention and vigilance (*sedation*, *somnolence*, and *distractibility*), impaired memory, and difficulty with complex mental functions. Patients treated with multiple AEDs (*polytherapy*), patients treated with high dosages, or patients who have high blood levels of AEDs are at the highest risk of cognitive deficits. However, some patients require high AED dosages or multiple AEDs to obtain seizure control, and these patients may tolerate high dosages or multiple AEDs without significant cognitive side effects. Everyone is different, and everyone responds a little differently to AEDs. In some people, the cognitive effects of AEDs can be severe enough to reduce a patient's perceived quality of life. Table 11.2, which identifies the adverse side effects of each of the AEDs you take, may help you and your doctor determine if you are suffering side effects from your AED.

Older AEDs

Carbamazepine (Tegretol, Carbatrol), phenytoin (Dilantin), valproate (Depakote), phenobarbital, and benzodiazepines are the "traditional" AEDs that have been used to treat epilepsy for many years. Cognitive side effects associated with these drugs in monotherapy are generally moderate but may be a problem for some. The cognitive effects of carbamazepine, phenytoin, and valproate appear to be very similar. In contrast, phenobarbital produces greater cognitive deficits than these other traditional AEDs.

Newer AEDs

Several but not all of the newer AEDs appear to have less cognitive effects than the older AEDs, although not all of the newer AEDs have been tested adequately for their cognitive effects. The best data for the newer AEDs exist for gabapentin (Neurontin) and lamotrigine (Lamictal). Both gabapentin and lamotrigine have few cognitive side effects and have been shown to have significantly less cognitive effects than the traditional AEDs and topiramate (Topamax). For example, both the traditional AEDs and topiramate can reduce verbal memory by 10% to 20%, but gabapentin and lamotrigine do not appear to adversely affect this type of memory in most people. Topiramate has been shown to have slightly more cognitive effects than the traditional AEDs and significantly more cognitive effects than gabapentin and lamotrigine. The cognitive effects of topiramate are increased if it is started rapidly, increased to high dosages, and used in polytherapy. These effects are also seen with other AEDs, but are more dramatic with topiramate. Nevertheless, topiramate is tolerated well in some patients, especially at lower dosages. Because other factors

TABLE 11.2
Adverse Events Profile

During the past 4 weeks, have you had any of the problems or side effects listed below? For each item, if it has always or often been a problem, circle 4; if it has sometimes been a problem circle 3; and so on. Please be sure to answer every item.

	Always or often a problem	Sometimes a problem	Rarely a problem	Never a problem
Unsteadiness	4	3	2	1
Tiredness	4	3	2	1
Restlessness	4	3	2	1
Feelings of aggression	4	3	2	1
Nervousness and/or agitation	4	3	2	1
Headache	4	3	2	1
Hair loss	4	3	2	1
Problems with skin, e.g., acne, rash	4	3	2	1
Double or blurred vision	4	3	2	1
Upset stomach	4	3	2	1
Difficulty in concentration	4	3	2	1
Trouble with mouth or gums	4	3	2	1
Shaky hands	4	3	2	1
Weight gain	4	3	2	1
Dizziness	4	3	2	1
Sleepiness	4	3	2	1
Depression	4	3	2	1
Memory problems	4	3	2	1
Disturbed sleep	4	3	2	1

contribute to the choice of AED—such as effectiveness in controlling seizures and other side effects (like weight gain)—topiramate will be the AED of choice for some patients.

Levetiracetam (Keppra) and tiagabine (Gabitril) seem to have few cognitive side effects. Oxcarbazepine (Trileptal) is better tolerated than several traditional AEDs, but has not been shown to have less cognitive effects than traditional AEDs in the few studies which assessed its effects. Not all of newer AEDs available in the United States have been tested for cognitive side effects, especially in populations at special risk, such as in children and the elderly.

Cognitive Effects of AEDs in Children and the Elderly

Children and the elderly are at special risk to suffer cognitive side effects from AEDs. The elderly are more susceptible to the cognitive effects of AEDs because they metabolize drugs differently and because drugs are more likely to impair their brain function. Children are potentially more susceptible because even modest effects of AEDs on attention and learning may be very important during early brain development. Unfortunately, no adequate studies have examined the cognitive effects of AEDs in both these age groups.

Several AEDs have been shown to cause greater cognitive side effects in the elderly. Benzodiazepines (Valium or diazepam) can impair cognitive abilities in the elderly and increase the risk of falling and hip fracture, presumably due to its effect on coordination. The cognitive side effects of carbamazepine, phenobarbital, phenytoin, and primidone (Mysoline) have been shown to be greater in elderly epileptic patients. Gabapentin and lamotrigine have been found to be better tolerated than carbamazepine in the elderly, primarily due to fewer side effects affecting the brain (cognitive problems, sedation, and dizziness). However, very few studies have directly compared the effects of different AEDs in the elderly.

Our information on the cognitive side effects of AEDs in children is also limited. Overall, the cognitive effects of carbamazepine, phenytoin, and valproate appear to be similar in children. Phenobarbital has been shown to cause adverse cognitive effects compared to *placebo* (a sugar pill) in children with *febrile* convulsions. Other studies have demonstrated greater adverse cognitive effects for phenobarbital compared to valproate. Despite the observation of differences in cognitive effects between some older and newer AEDs in adults, no studies have been done to measure the cognitive effects of the newer AEDs in children. Further, children may be at increased risk for long-term cognitive effects because of the possible effects of the AEDs on brain development (*neurodevelopment*). Since no long-term studies have been done, the risks of AEDs in children remain uncertain.

Exposure of the Fetus to AEDs

New concerns have been raised about the cognitive risk of AEDs in the fetus and in *neonates* (newborns). Experiments using newborn rats have shown that several older AEDs and phenobarbital cause long-term problems in cognition. Similar animal studies have found that phenytoin, phenobarbital, diazepam, clonazepam, and vigabatrin produce widespread loss of nerve cells in the brain. Topiramate and levetiracetam did not seem to produce these adverse effects in the newborn rat brain. (The other AEDs have not been tested in this way.)

These studies raise concern that similar effects may occur in newborn humans. Furthermore, since the developmental state of the neonatal rat brain is similar to the human fetal brain in the last few months of pregnancy, these studies also raise a concern that AED exposure in pregnant women may pose a risk for loss of brain cells in the unborn child. However, results in animals and in humans can differ as our information in humans is less complete and less certain.

Several recent studies in humans provide evidence that exposure to valproate during pregnancy poses a special risk. Although only a few studies in humans have examined the cognitive risk to the child of AED exposure during pregnancy, these also suggest a greater risk for valproate. One study has suggested a risk for phenobarbital exposure during pregnancy, and a few studies have suggested no increased risk exists for carbamazepine.

It's important to remember however that very few of these studies have been completed and much more information is needed for physicians to better advise women with epilepsy who want to become pregnant. *The majority of children born to epileptic women taking AEDs are normal*, despite the increased risk.

Women with epilepsy should not stop or decrease their AEDs without talking with their physician. The risks of the AED must be balanced against the risk of seizures. Women with epilepsy are at increased risk to die during pregnancy, primarily due to seizures—many of which occurred because the woman stopped or reduced her AED without talking with her physician (Chapter 8).

Summary

Patients with epilepsy frequently suffer from cognitive problems (see Table 11.1). Because epilepsy is caused by multiple diseases, the cognitive abilities of patients with epilepsy vary greatly. AEDs are the main treatment for epilepsy. The main concern in choosing an appropriate AED and dosage is control of seizures. However, another important concern is the effect of the AED on cognition, because adverse effects are common and may impair a patient's quality of life. Risk factors include polypharmacy and higher AED dosages or blood levels. Some AEDs pose an increased risk of cognitive side effects (phenobarbital). Several of the newer AEDs (such as gabapentin and lamotrigine) have been shown to have less cognitive effects that the traditional older AEDs. Our understanding of the cognitive effects of AEDs on children and the elderly is limited.

In patients who fail to achieve seizure control with AEDs, epilepsy surgery may offer their best hope of seizure freedom. Most patients can undergo epilepsy surgery without suffering new cognitive problems, but some risk exists (such as verbal memory decline after left temporal lobectomy). Studies done before the operation can largely define this risk, and thus help patients and their physicians make a decision based on the relative potential benefits and risks of the surgery.

COMMON PSYCHIATRIC DISORDERS IN EPILEPSY

For a long time, physicians have been aware of the fact that people with epilepsy are likely to experience various types of psychiatric disorders more frequently than the general population, as shown in Table 11.3. *Depression*, *anxiety disorders*, and *attention deficit disorders* (ADD) are the three most frequent psychiatric disorders identified in people with epilepsy. We'll take a closer look at these three problems here.

A common question asked by patients and physicians alike is to what degree is the epilepsy a cause of these psychiatric disorders. It's important to remember that seizure disorders are only one of many causes that contribute to the development of these three psychiatric disorders in people with epilepsy. And, we are far from having a complete understanding of *all* the causes of these psychiatric disorders in epilepsy.

In general, these three psychiatric disorders are more likely to be identified among people whose seizures are not well controlled. Unfortunately, patients are very often reluctant to let their doctor know about the presence of psychiatric symptoms, and consequently, they go untreated. This can have serious consequences on quality of life. Failure to seek treatment stems from various reasons, the two most frequent being: (1) a fear of being labeled "crazy" and (2) incorrectly believing that psychiatric symptoms are a "part of the epilepsy" and don't need special treatment.

Patients often say: "Wouldn't you be depressed or feel anxious if you were having epileptic seizures?" The fact is that, more often than not, these three psychiatric disorders are *not* due to a

---

TABLE 11.3
Prevalence Rates of Psychiatric Disorders in Epilepsy and the General Population

Psychiatric Disorder	Prevalence Rates	
	Epilepsy	General Population
Depression	11–50%	5–17%
Anxiety Disorders		
Generalized Anxiety Disorders	15–25%	5–7%
Panic Disorder	5–21%	0.5–3%
Attention Deficit Disorder (ADD)	12–37%	4–12%

reaction to having epilepsy. Therefore, any patient with psychiatric symptoms should be evaluated to determine the need for treatment. The good news is that effective treatment is available for depression, anxiety, and ADD in people with epilepsy.

Frequency

Table 11.3 compares the frequency of all three psychiatric disorders between people with epilepsy and the general population. Notice the higher frequencies among epilepsy patients. This does not mean that everyone with epilepsy will have these psychiatric problems. Also, people with milder forms of epilepsy are less likely to have psychiatric problems, or will have only mild symptoms. For example, the frequency of depression ranges from 10% to 50% among people with epilepsy; the lower percentages reflect the frequency of depressive disorders among patients with milder forms of epilepsy. This is also true for the other two disorders.

Depressive and anxiety disorders are the most frequently identified psychiatric disorders in adults with epilepsy, while ADD is the most frequent psychiatric disorder of children with epilepsy. This does not mean that depressive and anxiety disorders do not occur in children, or that ADD only occurs in children. In fact, all these disorders can occur both in adults and children, but their frequency has yet to be determined in these age groups.

Psychiatric Symptoms Related to Epilepsy

People with poorly controlled seizures may experience a *cluster* or group of psychiatric symptoms related in time to the occurrence of a seizure. Psychiatric symptoms can precede a seizure by a few hours to up to three days. We call these *preictal* symptoms. Psychiatric symptoms can also occur within a period of five days *after* a seizure, in which case we refer to them as *postictal* symptoms. Psychiatric symptoms may be the only or principal symptom of the actual seizure. We call these *ictal* psychiatric symptoms. Symptoms that occur independently of seizures are called *interictal* psychiatric symptoms.

Studies have shown that preictal and postictal psychiatric symptoms can include a wide variety of symptoms of depression (feeling sad, being unable to enjoy things, losing all hope, feeling helpless, crying constantly, and feeling guilty without a reason, wanting to be dead), symptoms of anxiety (worrying about everything without any apparent reason, feeling restlessness, inability to sleep, problems with concentration), as well as behavioral symptoms (irritability, impulsive and aggressive behavior, and hyperactivity). In the case of children, parents often report that they can predict when their child will have a seizure because she becomes more irritable and cranky, displays hyperactive behavior, and becomes more impulsive. Her behavior returns to "normal" after the seizure.

The postictal symptoms of depression, anxiety, and irritability can occur in up to 40% to 45% of people with poorly controlled seizures after more than 50% of their seizures. This means that these symptoms are a habitual occurrence. Often, these symptoms occur in the same patient. In contrast to preictal symptoms, patients often fail to make the connection between the occurrence of the seizure and postictal symptoms, because in the majority of cases these symptoms do not occur the same day of the seizure but rather one or two days later. Postictal symptoms of depression, anxiety, and behavior disturbances have been found to last from a few hours to several days, with an average duration of 24 hours. Clearly, the occurrence of pre- and postictal psychiatric symptoms can cause as much or more distress than the actual seizure to patients and family members alike!

Ictal psychiatric symptoms may occur in *simple partial seizures* and in some types of *temporal* or *frontal lobe epilepsies*. These symptoms are also known as *auras*. Feelings of fear or panic are the most frequently identified type of ictal psychiatric symptom, followed by depression. Often, auras are followed by a *complex partial seizure* or a convulsion, and hence the nature of these ictal psychiatric symptoms cannot be confused with a psychiatric disorder. On the other hand, patients experiencing only auras consisting of ictal panic can be erroneously diagnosed as suffering from panic attacks.

Depressive Disorders

Interictal depressive disorders are the most frequent psychiatric disorders in people with epilepsy. The most frequent types of depressive disorders include *major depression* and *dysthymic disorder*. The difference between major depression and dysthymic disorder is based largely on severity, persistence, and duration of symptoms.

Symptoms in both disorders may include combinations of depressed mood, inability to find any pleasure in any activity, feelings of worthlessness and guilt (without any apparent reason), feelings of helplessness and hopelessness, decreased ability to concentrate, recurrent thoughts of death, and problems with appetite resulting in weight loss or gain, changes in sleep causing insomnia or excessive sleep, slow thinking, agitation, and fatigue.

The diagnosis of a major depressive episode requires *at least 2 weeks* of either a depressed mood or inability to find pleasure accompanied by four or more of the additional symptoms listed occurring *every day* and lasting *the majority* of the day.

In contrast, dysthymic disorder is a more chronic but less intense situation, with symptoms present more days than not *for at least 2 years*.

People who have experienced one major depressive episode have a 50% chance of having more episodes. Those who have had two episodes have a 70% chance, and those who have experienced more than two episodes are likely to have recurrent major depressive episodes, unless they take medication to prevent it.

In addition, up to 50% of depressed people with epilepsy have an *atypical presentation* (unusual form) of their particular depressive disorder, one not usually seen in the general population. These atypical characteristics include the fact that their symptoms are recurrent but not continuous, with symptom-free periods that may last several days in duration. In addition, these patients report more apparent and frequent symptoms of irritability, poor frustration tolerance, and physical symptoms.

A large percentage of depressed people with epilepsy can also experience symptoms of anxiety or a full anxiety disorder and vice-versa. If your doctor is doing an evaluation to establish the presence of a depressive disorder, he also must evaluate you for the presence of symptoms of anxiety.

You should be aware of a disease called *manic-depressive illness* or *bipolar disorder* since it can present with major depressive episodes and it can occur in people with epilepsy more frequently than in the general population. A recent study showed that 12% of people with epilepsy had experienced symptoms of this condition at some point in their life. In bipolar disorder, the patient experiences recurrent major depressive episodes, followed by *manic* or *hypomanic episodes*. A manic episode consists of at least four of the following symptoms for a minimal period of at least 2 weeks: (1) inflated self-esteem or grandiosity, (2) decreased need for sleep, (3) more talkative than usual or pressured speech, (4) flight of ideas or racing thoughts, (5) distractibility, or (6) excessive involvement in pleasurable activities that have a high potential for painful consequences (such as unrestricted buying sprees, sexual indiscretions, etc.). The difference between manic and hypomanic episodes is also based on severity. A diagnosis of a hypomanic episode is reached after 4 days of a distinct and persistently elevated expansive or irritable mood associated with at least three of the above listed symptoms.

Depressive Disorders in Children with Epilepsy

It may be hard to recognize depressive disorders in children, both those with and without epilepsy. Children do not verbalize the "typical" symptoms of depression, such as "I am sad" or "I feel there is no hope for me." Instead, children tend to act out, become irritable or impulsive, and often display aggressive behavior at home and in school. They exhibit problems with concentration in school and are restless, which often leads physicians to make an erroneous diagnosis of ADD. Parents and physicians should suspect the possibility of a depressive disorder in a child who has: (1) a family history of depression or alcoholism in a first-degree relative, such as a parent or sibling; (2) problems with sleep, either difficulty falling asleep and waking up in the middle of the night, or excessive sleeping during the day; (3) changes in appetite, either as loss of appetite or excessive eating; (4) a tendency to withdraw from friends; (5) an avoidance or loss of interest in habitual or new recreational activities; and (6) a tendency of symptoms to recur with or without any apparent external reason following symptom-free intervals.

As in adults, depressive disorders in children are often associated with anxiety disorders or symptoms of anxiety.

Recognizing Depression in Epilepsy

It's important to recognize and treat depressive disorders early, because they may have a negative effect on quality of life. In fact, in people with persistent seizures, the presence of depression has a *worse* impact on their quality of life than the actual seizures themselves!

In addition, people with epilepsy have a greater risk of attempting or committing suicide than the general population. Clearly, an untreated depressive disorder can contribute to such higher suicidal risk.

Possible Causes of Depression in Epilepsy

Many things can contribute to depression in epilepsy. They include:

▶ A reaction to the multiple obstacles that people with epilepsy have to face, such as having to give up driving privileges (at least temporarily) and increased dependency on others for transportation, the stigma associated with having seizures in our society and the discrimination that often takes place at work and by peers, and the need to take daily medication, to name a few.

▶ Changes in the brain, consisting primarily of chemical and electrical changes caused by the actual seizure disorder. In addition, some of the areas of the brain that are affected by the epilepsy and the depressive disorder (in people without epilepsy) may be the same. For example, patients with temporal or frontal lobe epilepsy are more likely to experience depressive disorders. By the same token, people without epilepsy who suffer from major depression also may show abnormalities in their temporal and frontal lobes.

▶ A genetic predisposition. People with a family history of depression, especially in first-degree relatives (parents, siblings), may be at greater risk of experiencing depression associated with their epilepsy. It is important that you inform your doctor about a history of depression in your parents and close relatives, as certain AEDs can cause depression in patients with this type of family history. For example, if your mother suffered from depression, and you are started on a medication like phenobarbital, you are more likely to experience a depressive disorder.

An *iatrogenic process*. This is the occurrence of psychiatric complications directly related to the actual treatment of the seizure disorder with either antiepileptic medication or brain surgery (such as removal of the anterior part of the temporal lobe in patients with temporal lobe epilepsy). Table 11.4 shows the AEDs that have been found to frequently cause symptoms of depression or depressive disorders. When an AED causes symptoms of depression, lowering its dose may be enough to get rid of these symptoms. However, very often it is necessary to change the AED. On the other hand, in some patients with recurrent major depressive disorders or manic depressive illness, some AEDs, like carbamazepine (Tegretol), valproic acid (Depakote), and lamotrigine

---

TABLE 11.4
AEDs That Are More Likely To Cause Psychiatric Symptoms as Adverse Events

Symptoms of Depression/Anxiety	Behavioral Symptoms
Phenobarbital	Phenobarbital
Primidone (Mysoline)	Primidone
Clonazepam (Klonopin)	Clonazepam and other benzodiazepines
Felbamate (Felbamate)	Valproic acid (at high doses)
Topiramate (Topamax)	Topiramate
Levetiracetam (Keppra)	Levetiracetam
Zonisamide (Zonegran)	Gabapentin (in mentally retarded children)
	Lamotrigine (in mentally retarded children)

(Lamictal), can be very effective in preventing their recurrence. Stopping these AEDs in some people can actually cause psychiatric symptoms.

Treatment of Depression

Depressive disorders can be successfully treated with *antidepressants*. In addition, certain types of *psychotherapy* (or talk therapy), specifically cognitive behavior therapy *(CBT), may be very effective in helping patients* come out of a depressive episode. At times, a combination of antidepressant medication and CBT is recommended.

Because many physicians are afraid that antidepressant medication can worsen seizures, some have been reluctant to recommend this type of treatment. Nevertheless, studies have shown that the use of antidepressants known as *selective serotonin-reuptake inhibitors* (SSRIs) are safe in people with epilepsy and do not worsen seizures. There is no reason to withhold this type of treatment, above all in people with epilepsy who are experiencing a major depressive episode. SSRIs are also helpful in suppressing the symptoms of anxiety that very often accompany depressive episodes. Table 11.5 lists the most frequently used SSRIs in people with epilepsy

Antidepressant medication can be used safely in children and adolescents with depressive disorders and epilepsy. If this is necessary, however, they should be administered under the supervision of a child psychiatrist and not by the child's pediatrician.

As with any medication, SSRIs can potentially cause side effects. These include gastrointestinal symptoms (nausea, abdominal cramps, diarrhea, and heartburn), sedation or insomnia, and

TABLE 11.5
Efficacy of SSRIs and SNRIs in Primary Depression and Anxiety Disorders

Antidepressant Drug	Depression	Panic Disorder	Generalized Anxiety
Paroxetine (Paxil)	+	+	+
Sertraline (Zoloft)	+	+	
Fluoxetine (Prozac)	+	+	
Citalopram (Celexa)	+		
Escitalopram (Lexapro)	+	+	+

symptoms of sexual dysfunction (problems with erection or ejaculation). If any side effect occurs, inform your doctor. She may lower the dose and, if the symptoms do not disappear, change to another type of SSRI. You should not stop these medications abruptly, however, as you may experience some temporary nausea, headache, and flu-like symptoms.

Anxiety Disorders

As shown in Table 11.3, anxiety disorders are the second most common psychiatric disorder in people with epilepsy and they very often occur together with depressive disorders. The classification of anxiety disorders includes eight different types, of which *generalized anxiety disorder* and *panic disorder* are the two most frequent, both in the general population and in people with epilepsy. The other six disorders (agoraphobia without panic disorder, obsessive-compulsive disorder, social phobia, specific phobia, posttraumatic stress disorder, and acute stress disorder) may occur in people with epilepsy, but with a much lower frequency and will not be reviewed here.

In people with epilepsy, interictal panic and generalized anxiety disorders can be identical to those seen in the general population. Generalized anxiety disorder consists of constant uncontrollable worry on a daily basis, *of at least 6 months* duration, that is associated with at least three of the following six symptoms: restlessness, easy fatigability, decreased concentration, irritability, muscle tension, and sleep disturbances.

Panic disorder consists of recurrent panic attacks that are defined as "a discrete period" of intense fear or discomfort in which four or more of the following symptoms developed abruptly and reached a peak within 10 minutes: (1) fear of losing control or going crazy; (2) fear of dying; (3) palpitations or accelerated heart rate; (4) sweating; (5) trembling or shaking; (6) sensation of shortness of breath; (7) feeling of choking; (8) chest pain or discomfort; (9) nausea or discomfort in the abdomen; (10) feeling dizzy, unsteady, or faint; (11) feeling detached from oneself; (12) feelings of pins and needles; and (13) chills or hot flushes. It is not unusual for patients with panic disorders to avoid leaving the house or being left alone for fear of having a panic attack. When this happens, the patient is considered to have panic disorder with *agoraphobia*.

Patients with panic disorder may go through a period of several weeks to months with frequent panic attacks and then be free of panic attacks for prolonged periods. Also, panic attacks are not unusual when a patient is in the middle of a major depressive episode.

Ictal Panic and Its Differences with Interictal Panic Attacks

A feeling of panic can be the only expression of an aura or simple partial seizure. At times, patients with ictal panic have been erroneously diagnosed as having panic attacks. Taking a careful history of the event may avoid making such errors. The principal differences are: (1) ictal panics are short episodes lasting less than 30 seconds, while panic attacks last *at least* 10 to 20 minutes; (2) the intensity of the panic sensation is much less severe in ictal panic than in that of panic attacks and rarely do patients feel as if they are dying or going crazy; (3) the episodes of ictal fear are identical each time they occur, while such is not necessarily the case in panic attacks; and (4) patients with ictal fear may become confused or lose awareness of their surroundings if the seizure evolves to a complex partial seizure, while this does not happen in panic attacks.

Anxiety Disorders in Children with Epilepsy

In children, symptoms of anxiety usually are apparent in the form of *separation anxiety disorder*, which consist of the following symptoms: (1) fear (to the point of reaching a panic state) of staying alone in a room; (2) fear of going to bed alone or in a dark room; (3) constant worry about the whereabouts and welfare of the parents; (4) fear of something bad happening that may result in a separation from parents; and (5) complaints of a variety of physical symptoms such as headaches or stomachaches.

In its most severe form, separation anxiety can result in the child refusing to go to school. This is known as *school phobia*. When this happens, the child may wake early in the morning complaining about a variety of physical symptoms to avoid going to school, along with a long list of other reasons why he should stay at home. When school phobia occurs, immediate intervention by a child psychiatrist is advised, because the problem may become long-lasting.

The suspected causes of anxiety disorders in epilepsy are similar to the causes listed for depressive disorders.

Treatment of Anxiety Disorders in Epilepsy

As in the case of depressive disorders, treatment of anxiety includes the use of medication, CBT or other form of talk therapy, or a combination of both.

The same type of SSRI antidepressants listed for the treatment of depression are also very useful in the management of generalized anxiety disorder and panic disorder, at similar doses (see Table 11.5). In addition, *benzodiazepines* have been used for a very long time to treat anxiety disorders. The benzodiazepines include clonazepam and lorazepam, but these should only be given for a few weeks, as their efficacy may only last for a short time before fading.

ATTENTION DEFICIT DISORDERS

ADDs are the most frequent psychiatric disorder identified in children with epilepsy, although they occur in adults as well. ADDs can be divided into three principal categories: ADD predominantly with inattention, ADD predominantly with motor hyperactivity, and ADD with prominent presence of *both* inattention and motor hyperactivity. This last form is called *attention deficit hyperactivity disorder* (ADHD). The principal symptoms of interictal ADHD include motor hyperactivity, impulsive behavior, poor frustration tolerance, short attention span, and distractibility, which results in an inability to get organized in activities. Failure to concentrate makes learning difficult, and the child may appear forgetful and frequently lose things.

In the absence of motor hyperactivity and impulsive behavior, the child experiences all the problems derived from the poor concentration but no or fewer behavioral problems. With the exception of very severe forms of ADHD, symptoms often improve when the child is placed in a structured and quiet environment without too many things around him that may overstimulate or distract him. Children with ADHD often have associated learning disabilities and therefore they should be evaluated to identify their presence.

ADD in Adolescents and Adults with Epilepsy

Typically, when children with ADHD enter adolescence, their motor hyperactivity improves significantly but they may be left with problems of attention, impulsive behavior, and poor frustration tolerance. Adults with ADD complain primarily of difficulty concentrating, which results in problems with getting organized at their work and finishing their tasks, and may lead to constant job changes. In addition, they notice a propensity for being irritable and having a poor frustration tolerance.

ADHD can vary in severity from very mild to very severe. When mild, the symptoms may only be manifested as the child enters junior high or high school, where there is less structure and classes make more complex academic demands.

Causes of ADHD in Epilepsy

The suspected causes of ADHD in epilepsy include:

▶ Changes in the brain resulting in chemical and electrical changes caused by the epilepsy, or changes in the brain caused by the injury to the brain that caused the epilepsy. ADHD can be seen in all types of epilepsy, but more frequently in children with temporal and frontal lobe epilepsy. ADD can be seen frequently in children and adolescents who suffer from absence seizures and juvenile myoclonic epilepsy.

▶ A genetic predisposition. ADD can be inherited from one generation to the other.

▶ Iatrogenic causes. The antiepileptic medications that can cause symptoms of ADD are listed in Table 11.5.

Treatment of ADD

The treatment of ADD in patients with epilepsy includes medication and, in some cases, behavior and family therapy. Among the medications, drugs known as *central nervous system stimulants* are the most frequently used and are considered safe in children and adults with epilepsy. These include methylphenidate (Ritalin) and dextroamphetamine (Adderall). Until recently, the effect of these medications was of short duration, on the order of 3 to 4 hours, which required repeated doses. Most children were required to get their mid-day dose from the school nurse, which often can be very distressing and a cause of poor compliance. In the last decade, these medications have become available in formulations that last up to 12 hours. These *extended-release* formulations are now favored over the older ones.

Some physicians fear that the use of these medications can worsen seizures. This is not true; most pediatric neurologists and epileptologists believe that these drugs can be used safely in patients with epilepsy, and treatment should not be withheld because of such concerns.

The most frequent adverse events of central nervous system stimulants include decreased appetite, insomnia, abdominal pain, dry mouth, headaches, and nervousness. Approximately 10% of children with ADD may not be able to tolerate these drugs, becoming more irritable and moody instead. In these cases, the medication must be discontinued at once and another type of medication can be considered.

In addition to drug treatments, behavior therapy can be very helpful in training patients to develop strategies to control their impulsivity and poor frustration tolerance. Family therapy is often necessary to teach parents how to deal with these children.

SUMMARY

Patients with epilepsy are at a greater risk of experiencing depressive, anxiety, and attention deficit disorders than the general population. Early recognition of these psychiatric disorders is extremely important, as they can have a very negative impact on quality of life. While there may be an identifiable association between the seizure disorder and the development of any of these three psychiatric disorders, the causes of these psychiatric disorders in people with epilepsy are several, including a reaction to facing the obstacles of a life with seizures, changes in the brain resulting from the seizure disorder, a genetic predisposition, and side effects caused by AEDs. Nevertheless, not all the causes of these psychiatric disorders in epilepsy have been identified. People with epilepsy and any of these three psychiatric disorders must be evaluated for treatment, which is available, safe, and includes the use of medication, psychotherapy, or a combination of both.

FREQUENTLY ASKED QUESTIONS

Q Can AEDs impair my job performance?

A Most people taking AEDs can perform their job without problems, but AEDs can impair job performance in some people. Your risk may be increased if your job requires rapid motor responses, rapid processing of information, vigilance, or learning. Your risk may also be increased if you are taking multiple AEDs, higher dosages of AEDs with higher blood levels, or certain AEDs (such as topiramate or older AEDs, especially phenobarbital). If you have a concern, discuss it with your doctor.

Q I am worried about cognitive problems. What should I do, and what should I expect of my doctor?

A Talk with your doctor and let her know exactly what problems you are experiencing and how these problems are affecting your life. Factors that you and your doctor should consider as possibly contributing to your problem are listed in Table 11.1. If you are unsure if your AED(s) could be contributing to your problems, fill out the Adverse Events Profile in Table 11.2. If your total score is greater than 45, AED toxicity may be adversely impacting you. Your doctor may consider altering your AED treatment to reduce the dose, reduce the number of AEDs, or change to an AED with less cognitive side effects. Of course, these changes must take into account seizure control. Your doctor may also consider evaluations such as blood tests (such as AED blood levels, serum B_{12} level, thyroid tests), MRI, electroencephalogram (EEG), or formal neuropsychological testing) to detect abnormalities and direct your treatment.

Be aware that the underlying brain disorder that leads to epilepsy may also affect cognition. In fact, the size of the effect of the pre-existing brain disorder on cognition is usually larger than the effect of AEDs. However, the effect of AEDs can be significant, and AED effects can potentially be altered. Also, be aware that your mood can markedly affect your perception of your cognitive performance. In several studies, a patient's perception of their own cognitive abilities was more related to depressed mood than their actual cognitive performance. Further, depression can actually affect your attention and memory. Thus, your doctor may consider assessment and possible treatment for depression.

Q I am worried about cognitive problems in my child with epilepsy. What should I do?

A Many of the issues that you and your doctor should consider are the same as those discussed in Question 2 concerning this problem in the adult patient. However, this issue is complicated in children because their cognitive abilities are changing as they grow and because children may not be able to express their problems like an adult. School performance is an important factor that should be monitored. If you are concerned about your child's abilities, talk with your doctor. Your child may be eligible for Early Intervention Services. The Early Intervention Program for Infants and Toddlers with Disabilities of the Individuals with Disabilities Education Act (Part C) is available in all 50 states and seven territories of the United States. This program provides speech/language, occupational, and physical therapies to any child under the age of 3 who has a disability or significant delays in development. If your child has reached 3 years, she may be eligible for similar services through the Preschool Special Education Program in your local school district. Eligibility is determined by assessing your child's five skill areas: adaptive development, cognition, communication, physical development (gross and fine motor), and social/emotional development. Similar programs and therapies may also be available privately in your area.

Q I have suffered from epilepsy for several years, and my doctor has never asked me whether I was experiencing any symptoms of depression. Does that mean I do not have it or I do not need to worry about ever suffering from this disorder?

A The answer to this question is a definite No! Unfortunately, doctors may not inquire about the presence of depression or anxiety symptoms unless you appear sad and distressed during your medical visit or you verbalize symptoms of depression. Also, some doctors erroneously assume that experiencing symptoms of depression and anxiety is a "normal" reaction to having epilepsy and hence does not require special treatment. Yet, several causes may influence the development of depressive disorders, some of which may require an intervention. For example, if you are experiencing depressive symptoms caused by the AED that you are taking, you may be able to get rid of your symptoms by having your doctor lower the dose or change your medication. The important point to remember is that depression in people with epilepsy can disrupt life significantly, and the presence of symptoms of depression merits an evaluation to establish the need and type of treatment.

Q Can depressive and anxiety disorders interfere with my job performance?

A Absolutely! Depressive disorders can affect your job performance by interfering with your ability to think and to relate to others. For example, if you were to have a major depressive episode, you would experience slowed thinking and you would have difficulty concentrating and problems with remembering things. Because major depression causes irritability and poor frustration tolerance, you may end up arguing a lot with your co-workers and superiors, which could get you in trouble. You could potentially lose your job. If you are also experiencing symptoms of anxiety, you would have difficulty concentrating because of the constant worries and restlessness that would get in the way of your performance.

My Notes

12

TAKE CONTROL OF YOUR EPILEPSY

Your Rights, Government and Health Plans

Key Points

▶ The doctor-patient relationship stands in stark contrast to the adversarial relationships found in the areas of the law or when dealing with insurance companies.

▶ Both patients and doctors must treat each other with courtesy and respect.

▶ In the end, you are responsible for yourself. Your doctor is a source of information, but it is up to you to choose the option that is best for you.

▶ If you work with your PCP, and you continue to have seizures or side effects from medications, you should request a referral to see a neurologist who specializes in epilepsy.

▶ In general, it is unlawful for an employer to ask a job applicant about general medical problems, ask about a disability, or require a physical examination.

THE DOCTOR-PATIENT RELATIONSHIP

THE DOCTOR-PATIENT RELATIONSHIP demands commitment and compromise from both parties in order for treatment to be effective and efficient. Patients literally trust doctors with their lives. A doctor assumes that when a patient comes seeking care, he is telling the whole truth about his illness and that he wants to get better. Patients assume that their doctor will follow the highest standards of professional ethics and is genuinely interested in using medical expertise to help them get better. This arrangement creates a win-win situation that is gratifying to both patients and doctors alike: The patients receive good medical care and hopefully get better, and the doctors feels satisfied for helping patients and is usually paid for the services. This relationship between doctors and patients creates a special bond. So sacred is this trust, that many times, patients tell their doctors things about themselves that they would never tell anyone else, trusting that their doctors will safeguard this information and use it only to help heal them (Figure 12.1).

The doctor-patient relationship stands in stark contrast to the adversarial relationships found in the areas of the law or when dealing with insurance companies and the like. In these situations, the relationship begins with a dispute. One side presents an argument, and the other side presents a counter argument. In these disputes, lawyers are often involved. The role of the lawyer is to be an *advocate*: It is the lawyer's job to make the best case for his client, emphasizing the strong points and minimizing the weak points. Naturally, the other side is doing just the same, but selecting the presentation to favor its side of the dispute. A neutral third party, such as a judge or jury, weighs the evidence on both sides and concludes that one side wins and the other loses. These win-lose situations generally lead to hard feelings for at least half of the participants.

A patient has certain responsibilities to help make his health care better (see the Patient Bill of Rights, later in the chapter). Since most medical care takes place in a medical office, a patient should do certain things to make the visit more successful. The first is to tell your story as accurately as you can. Don't try to use medical words even if other doctors may have used them with you. Use your own words to tell your story. If you are asked a question that you

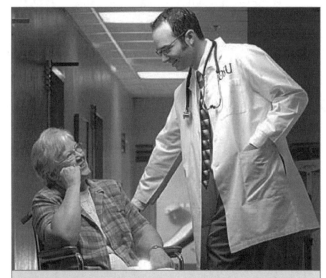

FIGURE 12.1
A good doctor-patient relationship is important.

can't answer, say so. Don't make up an answer to say what you think the doctor wants to hear. If your story is complicated, don't be afraid to write it down before you go to the doctor. Bring your medications with you in their prescription bottles to every visit. For people with epilepsy, bring a list of antiseizure medications you tried in the past and how your seizures responded, the maximum doses you took, and whether you had any side effects from the medications. Bring along the complete addresses of other doctors who have cared for you or to whom you want your records sent. If you can't describe what happens when you have a seizure, bring along someone who has seen your seizures, if you can. Try to obtain important records about your problem from other doctors and hospitals. Bring a list of questions you want to have answered. Don't be afraid to take notes, use a tape recorder, or ask someone else to sit in to take notes for you.

Your doctor has certain responsibilities at your office visit, too. Your doctor should greet you by name and listen attentively. Your doctor should also explain your diagnosis and give you some options to consider for diagnostic testing and treatment. In addition, your doctor should recognize that his role is to advise you with a set of sound medical choices and let you decide which one is best for you. After all, it is your life and you need to make informed decisions. If you are being given a medication, your doctor should tell you about the side effects and explain whether there are any drug interactions you need to be aware of. You should be given some idea about the likelihood of success in controlling your seizures. Similarly, you should be given detailed explanations about the risks and benefits of epilepsy surgery or implanted devices, if those are being considered for treatment options. Your doctor should also try to answer your questions in a language you can understand. You must be mindful that there may not be time to answer all of your questions, so try to ask the most important ones first. If your problem is complicated, expect having to make several visits in order to cover most of the questions you have.

Keep in mind that most doctors take care of about 2,000 patients, so try not to take up more than your fair share of their time during office visits, phone calls, and e-mails. If you are seeing a specialist for your epilepsy care, try to call him for issues only related to your epilepsy, and contact your primary care doctor for more general problems such as colds and refills of medications for other medical problems such as high blood pressure. If you do call for refills, have your pharmacy phone number ready before you call and also have a pen and paper handy in case you are given some new directions during the phone call.

Both patients and doctors must treat each other with courtesy and respect. Practice "The Golden Rule." Try to put yourself in the other person's position when you sense a conflict. Are you making a reasonable request? Avoid the temptation to place blame when things don't go as you expected.

Whenever we have an encounter with someone else, lots of unspoken communication takes place, in addition to the words we use. We automatically size each other up by eye contact, whether we stand or sit, by our dress, and in many other nonverbal ways. We have all met someone and come away feeling strongly positive or negative about the person we just met, perhaps only because that person had mannerisms that were similar to those of someone else about whom we also had strong feelings as well. These unconscious strong feelings are driven by hidden positive and negative bias that we all have based upon our own upbringing, sets of ideals for beauty, race, sex, social standing, and many other areas. Psychiatrists use the term *transference* to refer to these powerful emotions that patients have toward their doctors and *counter-transference* for the feelings that doctors have for their patients. No matter who we are, we get these feelings. By reflecting on these feelings, we can learn to know ourselves better and why we react the way we do under certain circumstances.

In the end, you are responsible for yourself. Your doctor is a source of information, but it is up to you to choose the option that is best for you. Therefore, listen to your doctor with an open mind. Speak up! Ask questions when you are uncertain. Only you know your own thoughts, so don't be afraid to express them. Reflect on your options but don't be paralyzed by indecision. Have the courage to make changes if you don't like how things are proceeding. That may mean having additional testing, trying a new medication, considering epilepsy surgery, or volunteering for a drug or device trial. It may mean seeking out a new doctor. If you have epilepsy, and you continue to have seizures, ask your doctor to refer you to a comprehensive epilepsy center. If your doctor resists, look up the names of some doctors at the closest epilepsy centers from the web sites of the Epilepsy Foundation, the American Epilepsy Society, or the National Association of Epilepsy Centers.

YOUR RIGHTS AS A PATIENT

In March 1998, President Clinton's Advisory Commission on Consumer Protection and Quality on the Health Care Industry, issued a report, "Quality First: Better Health Care for All Americans" that contained a Patients' Bill of Rights and Responsibilities (visit http://www.hcqualitycommission.gov/final/append_a.html). The Commission listed seven sets of rights and one set of responsibilities:

▶ The Right to Information. Patients have the right to receive accurate, easily understood information to help them make informed decisions about their doctors and other providers, hospitals and medical offices, and health plans.

▶ The Right to Choose. Patients have the right to a choice of health care providers that is sufficient to assure access to appropriate high-quality health care, including giving patients with serious medical conditions and chronic illnesses access to specialists.

▶ Access to Emergency Services. Patients have the right to access emergency health services when and where the need arises. Health plans should pay for services when patients go to any emergency department with acute serious symptoms "including severe pain" that "prudent laypersons" could reasonably expect would place their health at risk if they did not seek medical care.

▶ Being a Full Partner in Health Care Decisions. Patients have the right to fully participate in all decisions related to their health care. Consumers who are unable to fully participate in treatment decisions have the right to be represented by parents, guardians, family members, or others. Additionally, provider contracts should not contain any so-called "gag clauses" that restrict health professionals' ability to discuss and advise patients on medically necessary treatment options.

▶ Care Without Discrimination. Patients have the right to considerate, respectful care from all members of the health care industry at all times and under all circumstances. Patients must not be discriminated against in the marketing or enrollment or in the provision of health care services, consistent with the benefits covered in their policy and/or as required by law, based on race, ethnicity, national origin, religion, sex, age, current or anticipated mental or physical disability, sexual orientation, genetic information, or source of payment (Fig. 12.2).

▶ The Right to Privacy. Patients have the right to communicate with health care providers in confidence and to have the confidentiality of their individually identifiable health care information protected. Patients also have the right to review and copy their own medical records and request amendments to their records.

▶ The Right to Speedy Complaint Resolution. Patients have the right to a fair and efficient process for resolving differences with their health plans, health care providers, and the institutions that serve them, including a rigorous system of internal review and an independent system of external review.

▶ Taking on New Responsibilities. In a health care system that affords patients right and protections, patients must also take greater responsibility for maintaining good health. Greater involvement in their health care increases the likelihood of patients achieving the best outcomes and helps support quality improvement in a cost-conscious manner. According to the report, patient's responsibilities include:

▷ Take responsibility for maximizing healthy habits, such as exercising, not smoking, and eating a healthy diet.

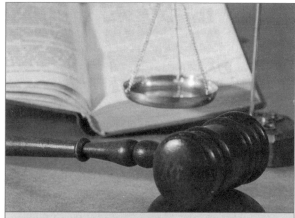

FIGURE 12.2
The law protects a patient's privacy.

▷ Become involved in specific health care decisions.

▷ Work collaboratively with health care providers in developing and carrying out agreed-upon treatment plans.

▷ Disclose relevant information, and clearly communicate wants and needs.

▷ Use the health plan's internal complaint and appeal processes to address concerns that may arise.

▷ Avoid knowingly spreading disease.

▷ Recognize the reality of risks and limits of the science of medical care and the human fallibility of the health care professional.

▷ Be aware of a health care provider's obligation to be reasonably efficient and equitable in providing care to other patients and the community.

▷ Become knowledgeable about health plan coverage and health plan options (when available) including all covered benefits, limitations, and exclusions, rules regarding use of network providers, coverage and referral rules, appropriate processes to secure additional information, and the process to appeal coverage decisions.

▷ Show respect for other patients and health workers.

▷ Make a good-faith effort to meet financial obligations.

▷ Abide by administrative and operational procedures of health plans, health care providers, and government health benefit programs.

▷ Report wrongdoing and fraud to appropriate resources or legal authorities.

The Health Insurance Portability and Accountability Act

The Health Insurance Portability and Accountability Act (HIPAA) Privacy Rule for the first time creates national standards to protect individuals' medical records and other personal health information. HIPAA was enacted by Congress in 1996 and came into effect in stages starting on April 14, 2003. While most of this section deals with the privacy aspects of the law, there are other sections to the law. One section protects workers and their families from losing health insurance coverage when they change or lose jobs. Another section establishes national standards for identification of health care providers, employers, hospitals, and health insurance plans and regulates how electronic transmission of health care information can occur so that security and privacy of the data is protected. HIPPA spells out how your health care record can be released and to whom it can be released. In general, the law gives patients more control over their data than they had before. The details of the national standards can be found at the Health and Human Services Office of Civil Rights web site, http://www.hhs.gov/ocr/hipaa/.

HIPAA affects patients in many ways. It generally gives patients the right to examine and obtain a copy of their own health records and request corrections. It sets up rules for safeguarding the privacy of your medical records and details the penalties that can be imposed if privacy is not maintained. It spells out how some aspects of your records can be released, such as in matters related to protecting public health, but generally allows you to find out who was given this information and when it was given. It gives you the ability to limit the release of some aspects of your medical records.

For parents, it generally allows parents and guardians to have access to the medical records of their minor children as long as no other laws cover release of the information. For example, parents would not have access if the court ordered the child to undergo some medical treatment, if the minor consents to care that does not require parental approval, or if the parent agrees that the minor may have a confidential relationship with the provider. Even in these situations, there may be some situations in which parents will be allowed access to some of the information. On the other hand, the minor's privacy may be protected in certain circumstances, such as if the provider believes that the child might be subject to domestic violence or abuse if the information became known to the parent. The HIPAA Privacy Rule does not change the rules regarding a child's ability to be treated without parental consent.

YOUR INSURANCE COMPANY

Insurance companies generally sell policies to employers, who then provide this insurance to their employees and their families. Every policy is a contract—an agreement that certain medical services will be paid for and others will not. The services that the policy will pay for are called *covered benefits*. A covered benefit may be fully paid by the policy, or only a portion may be paid with the expectation that you will be responsible for paying the remaining amount. The part that you pay is called a *deductible*. Many policies have a number of fixed deductibles where you might be required to pay $5, $10, $50, or more for certain services. Other policies may require you to pay a certain percentage of the total charge for the same services. It is common for policies to have a mixture of both types of deductibles.

SECOND OPINIONS

An important element of health is to feel that you have some control over your destiny and to take steps to do those things that are important to controlling your health. When you take steps to positively influence your health, called *self-management*, you will find that your self-esteem will improve and you will feel more confident in your abilities to handle the world around you. One word of caution—many insurance plans will not pay for a "*second opinion*" visit except as a required prelude to certain elective procedures such as operations for low back pain. When you are seeking the opinion of a new doctor, such as an epilepsy specialist, you are actually asking for a *consultation*. If your doctor will not give you a referral for a second opinion, try to make an appointment as a "new patient." Each of these terms—second opinion, consultation, and *new-patient visit*—requires a different billing code and has a different charge for the visit. As a rule, second opinions have the most expensive charges, and new-patient visits have the least expensive charges.

One tricky area of self-management happens when you feel that the care you are getting may not be the best for you. Perhaps you continue to have seizures despite doing everything your doctor has recommended. Maybe you feel that the doctor is not really listening to you. The goal of epilepsy treatment is to be free of seizures and free of side effects. If you continue to have seizures despite working with your doctor for many months, or if you have side effects from medications that interfere with doing the things that you want to do, you should consider trying a new approach. The first step if you have a doctor that you like is to talk to her about whether it is time to try something different. Ask about diagnostic tests that might be done, such as epilepsy video-electrocephalogram (V-EEG) monitoring. Ask about new medications or treatments, such as surgery, that might help you.

DEALING WITH YOUR HMO

Two major types of insurance policies are available for health care. The traditional health care insurance policy, called *indemnity insurance*, provides payments for health care claims that are submitted by any doctor or hospital you use to provide health care. These payments are determined by your contract. With indemnity insurance, you are free to choose any doctor or hospital that has a contract with the health plan. If you choose other doctors or hospitals, you may have to pay for your care initially and then submit the payments to your insurance company for reimbursement. Indemnity insurance typically gives you the greatest choice of where you can receive medical care. One criticism of indemnity care is that this type of insurance provides a "blank check" to health care providers and leads to spending money on unneeded services and procedures since the more the doctor does, the greater the income to the practice. Because of emphasis on payment for expensive tests and treatments, indemnity insurance is the most expensive type of health insurance. Another criticism of this type of insurance is that patients with complicated problems end up with many teams of doctors who are looking out for only a small part of the patient's problems—no one is able to see the big picture and sort out what may be best overall for a patient.

The other major model of health care is called a *Health Maintenance Organization* or *HMO*. The HMO philosophy is based upon the idea that an organized system of health care that emphasizes preventive services (such as vaccines and regular checkups) will provide a higher level of health care at a lower overall cost than traditional indemnity insurance. A central part of HMO plans is the assignment of each patient to a *primary care provider* or *PCP* who is responsible for oversight of that patient's care. The PCP is usually a physician but sometimes may be a physician's assistant or nurse practitioner. In most HMOs, a PCP will have about 2,000 patients to care for. This is known as a *panel*. The PCP is also known as the *gatekeeper*, because all your health care is funneled through that individual. Each physician's panel is reviewed by HMO administrators to determine that the physician is providing the proper amounts of preventative care, referrals to specialists, and mix of medications. These audits typically track services as the total performed per member per month (PMPM). These ratios are compared to other PCPs in the same plan and often to other HMOs across the country to see how your doctor measures up. HMOs typically choose target goals for many services, setting the best HMO performance as benchmarks. Many national organizations compare HMOs on how they measure up to the benchmarks. Much of this data is published on the Internet. A typical example of this can be found at the NCQA web site, http://www.ncqa.org/.

In a typical HMO, you will need a referral from your PCP to see any other doctor, such as a neurologist. In practice, many HMOs will allow you to see a limited set of other specialty services, such as eye care services or obstetrics and gynecological services, without a referral. The theory behind this is that your PCP knows you best of all and can coordinate your health care needs in an organized fashion. In HMO plans, a large number of doctors and hospitals are gathered together to form a *network* to provide for care of the members. All your care will be given by members of this network unless you receive special permission to go "outside of the network" for a service not provided by the HMO.

In the HMO model, the network is provided with a fixed annual sum of money for each member of the network to pay for all the health care costs of the HMO's subscribers. The doctors in an HMO do not receive any extra money for additional services, so their incentive should be to do what is best for the patient. In practice, this can be an incentive to do as little as possible, since internal accounting practices track the costs of all services and deduct that from the general pool. In for-profit HMOs, any unspent money left over at the end of the year is paid out to stockholders and to the doctors as profits and bonuses. In a non-profit HMO, the need to generate a profit on health care is not an issue, so the money set aside for profit in a for-profit HMO can be applied to patient care. For many patients, health care in the best non-profit HMOs is excellent.

There are some variations on the HMO model such as *Preferred Provider Organizations* (PPO) and *Point of Service* (POS) plans that operate similar to HMOs but give the consumer more choice in selection of doctors. In these plans, consumers are able to choose providers outside of the list of doctors in the plan, but must pay more for the services from these doctors.

HMOs function very well for members with healthy families, since many routine services such as checkups and vaccinations are encouraged and often provided free of charge. The HMO system can be much more difficult for people with some chronic illnesses. Some PCPs may be reluctant to refer you to a specialist since there may be pressure on your PCP to limit referrals to keep down costs. The specialist that you may be referred to may be only allowed to see you for a few visits or perhaps only a single visit. The specialist may not be allowed to order any tests, and the medical or surgical options covered may be limited as well. In addition, the specialist that you are referred to may not be the best one in your region for your particular problem because that doctor might be out of network.

If you have a condition such as epilepsy, your goal should be to have "no seizures and no side effects from treatment." If you work with your PCP, and you continue to have seizures or side effects from medications, you should request a referral to see a neurologist who specializes in epilepsy. If you are referred to a general neurologist, you should give that doctor a reasonable amount of time, say 3 to 6 months, to control your epilepsy. If you continue to have seizures or side effects, then you should ask your PCP to refer you to an epilepsy specialist, also known as an *epileptologist*. Most epilepsy specialists practice in epilepsy centers with other specialists and offer special services such as epilepsy surgery and opportunities to volunteer for research with new medications or new devices. In addition, epilepsy centers have social workers, nurses, and psychologists who also specialize in epilepsy care and may provide you with the help you need. You can find a listing of most of the epilepsy centers in the United States by checking the web site of the National Association of Epilepsy Centers, www.naec-epilepsy.org. Ask your doctor to refer you to a member of the NAEC if your seizures remain uncontrolled.

If your doctor does not give you a referral to the specialist you would like to see, you have some options. Fortunately, HMO plans all have appeals processes for its members. You have the right to petition the HMO for a referral. If you are unsuccessful in getting the referral you wish, call the HMO central administration office and ask to speak to the person who handles appeals for referrals. You may need to fill out some forms. You need to be assertive and explain clearly why you want to be referred and to whom. If you have epilepsy, you should not accept anything less than "no seizures, no side effects" until you have gotten a thorough evaluation by a specialist, including diagnostic tests such as a video-EEG monitoring of your typical seizures and appropriate diagnostic tests such as a high-quality MRI. If you are turned down by the appeals board, do not hesitate to ask your employer or your union to help you with your appeal. After all, your employer is paying a lot of money for your health care, and the company deserves to get its money's worth for the premiums it pays. If all else fails, you can appeal to the state insurance commissioner.

GETTING YOUR MEDICATIONS

Anticonvulsant drugs are the mainstay of treatment for people with epilepsy. About a dozen major drugs are used to treat people with epilepsy, and a number of minor ones as well. Anticonvulsant drugs vary considerably in price, ranging from pennies a tablet for phenobarbital to more than $3 a tablet for some of the newest medications. All insurance plans have many policies on prescription drug coverage. They do this because the drug coverage benefit is purchased by a company for the benefit of its employees. Employers try to balance the cost of the drug benefit with what is covered. Because there are many thousands of different drug benefits plans, only a few of the common features will be addressed.

Most insurance plans have a list of drugs that are covered under the policy. The listing of those covered drugs is called the *formulary*. The drug formulary is typically divided into two or three tiers of drugs for prescription medications. A typical three-tier plan may charge you $10 per prescription for drugs on a *preferred* drug list, such as first-line generic medications. The $10 is called your *co-pay*. The drugs in the first tier are selected because they are drugs that have been shown to be helpful for large numbers of patients or conditions, with a track record of safety and low cost. The second tier of drugs contains those that may have more limited uses, more side effects or safety issues, and/or higher cost. In a three-tier prescription benefit, the second tier, or *second-line drugs* will often have a co-pay of $15 to $30 or more. The most expensive drugs are usually found in the third tier, although some less expensive drugs that may be particularly difficult to use because of side effects or interactions with other medications may be found in this tier as well. You may have a fixed co-payment for third-tier drugs, say $50, or you may have to pay a certain percentage of the total cost of the prescription, which could range between 10% and 50% or more of the total cost.

Many policies will use mail-in pharmacies to deliver your medications. These prescriptions are usually for a 90-day supply. For drugs dispensed at your local pharmacy, most companies will permit your doctor to write prescriptions for as much as a 30- to 35-day supply. The insurance company charges are determined by the details of the policy. Doctors are bound to follow the rules of the contract you have, so please do not ask your doctor to violate the rules of contract by prescribing more medication than is specified in the contract, regardless of whether you are getting your prescriptions filled at a pharmacy or by mail. By doing so, you are asking your doctor to commit fraud.

MEDICARE PRESCRIPTION DRUG BENEFIT, MEDICARE PART D

Some people with epilepsy do not have prescription drug coverage benefits. Until 2006, this was the situation for Medicare, but a new prescription drug benefit will make a major difference to people on Medicare and many of those on Medicaid as well. The 2003 *Medicare Modernization Act* (MMA) added a new voluntary prescription drug benefit, Medicare Part D. Details can be found at the Medicare web site, http://www.medicare.gov/ medicarereform/drugbenefit.asp. For people without a computer connection, you can call the 24-hour-a-day hotline, 1-800-MEDICARE (1-800-633-4227).

The Medicare prescription drug benefit has a complicated formula that requires a monthly premium of about $37 for 2006 and a $250 yearly deductible for medication. You will also pay part of the cost of each prescription. Expect to pay about 25% of the cost for the first $2,250 spent on drugs (about $525). You will pay 100% of the charges from $2,250 to $5,100 ($2,850) and then 5% coverage of expenses greater than $5,100 per year. Special help is available for low-income patients. If you make less than $11,000 (single) or $23,000 (married), you may be eligible for additional aid. In addition, each Medicare enrollee must pick a Prescription Drug Plan to provide their drugs.

In October 2005, Medicare beneficiaries were mailed information on their choices. Medicare recipients were able to sign up for the plan of their choice starting on November 15, 2005, with prescriptions filled as of January 1, 2006. If you signed up after January 1, 2006, your coverage started on the first day of the next following month. If you signed up after May 15, 2006, your monthly premium may be higher than the average of $37.

For patients covered by Medicare and state Medicaid—the so-called "dual eligibles"—your state no longer provides medication coverage as of January 1, 2006. These patients have been transferred from their state plans to one of the Medicare plans available in their state on January 1, 2006. If they did not choose a plan by then, they were assigned to a plan. Dual-eligible patients will be given aid to cover some of the costs of the prescriptions.

Medicare enrollees have a choice of prescription drug plans to choose from as the provider of coverage. Each state has at least 10 plans. The listings for each state and the costs are available at the Medicare web site, http://www.medicare.gov/medicarereform/map.asp. Medicaid-Medicare dual eligibles usually are limited in their choice of the prescription drug plans available in their state.

Each prescription drug plan has a formulary guided by the model formulary developed in 2004 by the United State Pharmacopoeia (www.usp.org). At this time, the formulary for each provider is not listed. Fortunately, anticonvulsant drugs are widely available because of the successful advocacy of the Epilepsy Foundation, the National Association of Epilepsy Centers, and the American Academy of Neurology. The anticonvulsant drugs are classed based upon the major mechanism of action: sodium channel inhibition, GABA augmentation, glutamate reduction, calcium channel modification, and others. One important exception is that the Medicare Modernization Act prohibits reimbursement for controlled substances. Several anticonvulsant drugs are classified as Schedule IV controlled substances and are not covered under Medicare Part D. The noncovered drugs are phenobarbital, diazepam (Valium, Diastat), lorazepam (Ativan), clonazepam (Klonopin), midazolam (Versed), and clorazepate (Tranxene). All these drugs are available as inexpensive generic drugs, with the exception of the Diastat formulation of diazepam.

DRIVING

With the exception of residents of a few large cities, driving a car is the major mode of travel for Americans. Thus, for people with epilepsy, not being able to drive is one of the greatest frus-

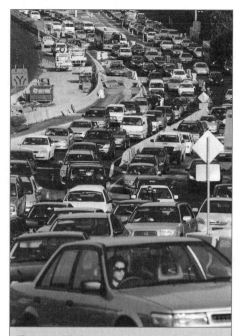

FIGURE 12.3
For many Americans, driving means independence.

trations they face. Not only is it inconvenient, it reinforces the notion that they are not independent adults. Each state sets regulations about driving in that state. The Epilepsy Foundation keeps track of the regulations for each state and posts them on their web site, www.epilepsyfoundation.org (Table 12.1). Most states make additional restrictions for driving commercial vehicles. Fortunately, only a few states require physicians to report patients who have had seizures to the state department of motor vehicles (Figure 12.3). In addition, the Federal Motor Carrier Safety Administration has issued recommendations for medical examiners to determine a driver's medical qualifications for driving vehicles for interstate commerce. These guidelines are spelled out in Section 391.41 of the Federal Motor Carrier Safety Regulations (FMCSRs), http://www.fmcsa.dot.gov/rulesregulations/administration/medical.htm. This regulation is advisory for medical personnel doing certification examinations for interstate commercial driver's licenses. These regulations are considered the minimum restrictions, since examiners may hold a driver to a higher standard.

Section 391.41(b)(8) deals with epilepsy. In this section, it states that a driver with a clinical diagnosis of epilepsy and recurrent seizures of any cause or one who is taking antiseizure medication should never be certified. A driver who has had a single unprovoked seizure or episode of fainting may be certified, but only if the driver is not taking medications and has been free of seizures *off medication* for 5 years following the single seizure. For people with multiple seizures, the driver must be free of seizures for 10 years *off medication* from the last seizure to qualify to drive. Fever seizures of childhood are not disqualifying. All questionable spells require a waiting period of 6 months off medication, followed by a complete neurologic examination to be cleared to drive. For people with acute provoked seizures, such as a seizure caused by drug reaction or an acute metabolic disturbance, the individual must wait until he has fully recovered, has no residual complications, and is not taking antiseizure medication.

WORKING

Patients with epilepsy are well aware of the difficulties they face when trying to get or keep a job. According to the Epilepsy Foundation, the rate of unemployment for people with epilepsy is 25%. How much of this is due to discrimination is difficult to determine. Most of this discrimination is hidden because there are laws against discriminating against people with disabilities.

A number of federal laws protect against discrimination due to epilepsy. They can be found at http://www.dol.gov/compliance/topics/hiring-disabilities.htm. Title I of the Americans with Disabilities Act (ADA) prohibits employers with 15 or more employees—including state and local governments, employment agencies, and labor organizations—from discriminating in employment against qualified individuals with disabilities. Title II of the ADA prohibits state and local governments from discriminating against qualified individuals with disabilities in programs, activities, and services. The ADA is primarily enforced by the Equal Employment Opportunity Commission (EEOC), an independent federal agency. Section 503 of the Rehabilitation Act of 1973 requires federal contractors and subcontractors to employ and advance in employment qualified individuals with disabilities, and it prohibits discrimination against such individuals. Section 504 of the Rehabilitation Act of 1973 prohibits discrimination on the basis of status as a qualified individual with a disability in programs and activities that receive certain federal funding. Some other protections from discrimination are found in Section 188 of the Workforce Investment Act of 1998 (WIA).

The Fair Labor Standards Act (FLSA) establishes the federal minimum wage and overtime pay requirements. This law also contains a provision allowing for the employment of individuals with disabilities at special minimum wages. This law governs how much people employed in sheltered workshops are paid. Generally, they must be paid at a rate relative to what a nondisabled person would be paid for similar quality and amount of work.

People with epilepsy and a history of epilepsy are specifically mentioned as having a qualified disability in the ADA and Section 503. These regulations also protect people with epilepsy who have recovered from their disability but who may face job discrimination because of their past medical records or because employers may incorrectly think of them as disabled when they are not. Of course, the person applying for a job must have the necessary education, skills, or other functions of the job. Such a person is called a *qualified individual* in the ADA. However, the employer and the employee both must make *reasonable accommodations* if the disability interferes with performing essential features of the job. Three separate categories of reasonable accommodations exist: (1) modifications to the job-application process that enables disabled individuals to be considered for jobs; (2) accommodations on the job; and (3) accommodations made to allow disabled individuals to enjoy equal benefits and privileges of employment.

An employer must make accommodations unless the accommodation poses an "undue burden" to the employer. Just what an "undue burden" is depends upon a number of factors such as the size of the company, the cost and extent of the accommodation, and so on. The employer is not required to substantially change the job requirements. The accommodation must be tailored to the individual and should be seen as a give-and-take transaction between the employer and the employee, both working in good faith to find an acceptable accommodation that permits the employee to perform the essential features of the job. Sometimes, the patient's physician can play an important role in finding acceptable accommodations. If employees are having problems meeting job demands, they should be proactive and raise the issue with their employers, rather than wait until disciplinary actions start before they complain. If the employee and employer have difficulty arriving at a satisfactory accommodation, the Job Accommodation Network (JAN) may be helpful. Their web site is http://janweb.icdi.wvu.edu and their phone number is 1-800-526-6080.

MEDICAL EXAMINATIONS AND PRE-EMPLOYMENT INQUIRIES

In general, it is unlawful for an employer to ask a job applicant about general medical problems, ask about a disability, or require a physical examination. The employer is allowed to ask an applicant if he has any limitations about performing the job with or without accommodation. The employer may ask an applicant to describe or demonstrate how to perform the essential duties of the job either with or without accommodation. After making an offer to hire an applicant, the employer may require a physical examination and may make the final job offer conditional on passing the physical examination only if all other applicants for the same job undergo similar examinations.

If you feel that you have been discriminated against, you must file a complaint with the nearest Equal Employment Opportunity Commission office within 300 days from the date of the alleged discrimination. The phone number is 1-800-649-4000 (voice) or 1-800-669-6820 (TDD). If the EEOC dismisses the complaint or fails to take action within 180 days, the EEOC will issue a right-to-sue letter. The individual then has 90 days to file a lawsuit. The Epilepsy Foundation has the Jeanne A. Carpenter Legal Defense Fund to help people who feel that they have been discriminated against. They have a list of lawyers across the country who can help you with your problem, in addition to the help that they can provide. They can be contacted at 1-800-EFA-1000 or at http://www.epilepsylegal.org. For general legal information about epilepsy in the workplace, please visit http://www.epilepsyfoundation.org/answerplace/Legal.

Unfortunately, some recent Supreme Court rulings have made it more difficult to claim discrimination under the ADA. The Court has ruled that you must prove a substantial disability. The Court has said that a condition that is controlled by medication does not qualify for ADA protection unless substantial disability continues to exist. For example, a woman with epilepsy may have found that medication fully controls her seizures but the side effects of the medication may slow her thinking to the point that she may have difficulty working at the same rate as other employees. She may ask for accommodation under the ADA in these circumstances. There are a number of challenges to the ADA in the courts at this time. It is not clear how the ADA will be altered, if at all, by these cases. The Epilepsy Foundation is following these cases carefully and will keep updated information at their web site.

SEIZURES AND SHORT-TERM DISABILITY FROM WORK

Patients often come to a clinic or call after having had a seizure and want to have a letter to return to work. Physicians are often faced with a dilemma when deciding when (or if) a patient can return to work and what kind of job restrictions are necessary to protect the patient and his co-workers should another seizure occur. If the patient's job involves driving, then the rules are clear-cut and the patient will not be able to work at his usual duties until driving privileges are restored. Unless suitable alternative work can be arranged, this can mean an extended time off work or life-long loss of job duties for commercial drivers, as detailed in the sections earlier in this chapter. For people with sedentary jobs, breakthrough seizures may not pose much of a problem at all. However, there are many people, particularly those in manufacturing or construction fields, for whom break-through seizures produce major problems in deciding when it is safe to return to work. If alternative duties are available that can be safely performed even if the patient has another seizure, then the patient can promptly return to work. If not, a common approach of many physicians is to use the driving regulations for their state and take the time that a license is suspended to be a suitable proxy for the time needed to be off work. The reasoning behind such actions is that, if the state has determined that the seizure-free period is sufficient for returning to driving, then it must be safe for returning to most jobs as well. Most employers feel comfortable with this approach as well.

My Notes

_____

_____

_____

_____

_____

_____

_____

Table 12.1 Driving Restrictions for Epilepsy Patients by Individual States

State	Seizure Free Period (months)	Physicians Report Required
Alabama	6*	
Alaska	6	
Arizona	3*	
Arkansas	12	
California	3, 6, or 12*	Yes
Colorado	None	
Connecticut	None	
Delaware	None	Yes
District of Columbia	12	
Florida	6* Upon Recommendation	
Georgia	6	
Hawaii	6*	
Idaho	6* Upon Recommendation	
Illinois	None	
Indiana	None	
Iowa	6*	
Kansas	6*	
Kentucky	3	
Louisiana	6* Dr. Statement Required	
Maine	3*	
Maryland	3	
Massachusetts	6*	
Michigan	6	
Minnesota	6*	
Mississippi	12	
Missouri	6* Upon Recommendation	

TABLE 12.1 Driving Restrictions for Epilepsy Patients by Individual States

State	Seizure Free Period (months)	Physicians Report Required
Montana	None* Upon Recommendation	
Nebraska	3	
Nevada	3	Yes
New Hampshire	12	
New Jersey	12	Yes
New Mexico	12*	
New York	12*	
North Carolina	6 to 12	
North Dakota	6* Restricted License at 3	
Ohio	None	
Oklahoma	6	
Oregon	6*	Yes
Pennsylvania	6*	Yes
Puerto Rico	None	
Rhode Island	18*	
South Carolina	6	
South Dakota	6 to 12*	
Tennessee	6 with Medical Form	
Texas	6 Upon Recommendation	
Utah	3	
Vermont	None	
Virginia	6*	
Washington	6*	
West Virginia	12*	
Wisconsin	3 with Medical Form	
Wyoming	3	

* Discuss with your Physician

Information up to date as of May 2007

APPENDIX

Resources

PHARMACEUTICAL AND MEDICAL DEVICE COMPANIES

Medications, Web Sites, and Contact Information

Abbott Laboratories (Depacon, Depakote). http://www.abbott.com, (847) 937-6100

Cephalon (Gabitril). http://www.cephalon.com, (800) 896-5855

Cyberonics, Inc. (Vagal Nerve Stimulator). http://www.cyberonics.com, (888) 867-7846

Glaxo Smith Kline (Lamictal). http://www.gsk.com, (888) 825-5249

Novartis (Tegretol, Trileptal). http://www.pharma.us.novartis.com, (888) 669-6682

Ortho-McNeil Pharmaceuticals (Topamax). http:/ /www.ortho-mcneil.com, (800) 526-7736

Pfizer (Cerebyx, Dilantin, Neurontin, Zarontin, Lyrica). http://www.pfizer.com, (866) 706-2400

Roche Laboratories (Klonopin). http://www.rocheusa.com, (973) 235-5000

Sanofi-Aventis (Mebaral). http://www.sanofi-aventis.us/, (800) 981-2491

Shire (Carbatrol). http://www.shire.com/shire, (484) 595-8800

UCB Pharma (Keppra, Keppra XR, Vimpat). http://www.ucb-group.com/, (770) 970-7500

Med Pointe (Felbatol). http://www.medpointepharma.com/, (732) 564-2200

Valeant (Diastat, Mysoline). http://www.valeant.com, (800) 511-2120

DIRECTORY OF PRESCRIPTION DRUG PATIENT ASSISTANCE PROGRAMS

Abbott (Depakote)
200 Abbott Park Road D31C, AP52, Abbott Park, IL 60064
(800) 222-6885

Cephalon (Gabitril)
P.O. Box 4280, Gaithersburg, MD 20885-4280
(866) 209-7589

EISAI Inc. (Banzel)
100 Tice Boulevard, Woodcliff Lake, NJ 07677
(866) 728-4368

Glaxo Smith Kline (Lamictal)
P.O. Box 29038, Phoenix, AZ 038-9038
(866) 728-4368

Med Pointe (Felbatol)
P.O. Box 1001, Cranbury, NJ 08512
(800) 678-4657

Novartis (Tegretol, Tegretol-XR, Trileptal)
P.O. Box 66556, St. Louis, MO 63166-6556
(800) 277-2254

Ortho-McNeil (Topamax)
P.O. Box 22187, Charlotte, NC 28222-1857
(800) 652-6227

Pfizer (Dilantin, Neurontin, Zarontin, Lyrica)
P.O. Box 66585, St. Louis, MO 63166-6585
(800) 707-8990

Roche (Klonopin)
340 Kingsland Street, Nutley, NJ 07110
(800) 443-6676

Shire (Carbatrol)
P.O. Box 698, Sommerville, NJ 08876
(866) 325-8224

UCB Pharma (Keppra, Keppra XR, Vimpat)
1950 Lake Park Drive, Smyrna, GA 30080
(800) 477-7877 (option 7)

Valeant (Diastat, Mysoline)
P.O. Box 4008, Clinton, NJ 08809
(800) 511-2120

HOME SAFETY CHECKLIST

Kitchen, Cooking, Barbecue

▶ Ask someone to assist you when starting open fires, grills, etc.
▶ Avoid boiling or frying in large pots and pans.
▶ Avoid using a gas stove and cook with an electric or microwave oven.
▶ Use rear burners when cooking.
▶ Avoid using an electric knife.
▶ Use oven mitts.
▶ Use a car to transport hot food on wheel from the stove to the table.
▶ Install heat control devices in kitchen faucets to prevent scalding.
▶ Use plastic containers rather than glass.

Bathrooms

▶ Never lock bathroom door.
▶ Take showers rather than baths.
▶ If taking a bath only use a few inches of water.
▶ Use a handheld shower head and sit while showering.
▶ Install heat-control devices in bathrooms to prevent scalding.
▶ Shave with an electric shaver.

General

▶ **Do not hunt, handle firearms, or use any potentially harmful objects.**
▶ Try to live in a one floor dwelling and avoid using stairs.
▶ Use an iron that shuts off automatically and avoid using a curling iron.

▶ Keep a protective screen in front of the fireplace.

▶ Avoid exposed heaters.

▶ Do not smoke cigarettes.

▶ Install smoke alarms.

▶ Check in with a friend or family member at least once a day.

▶ Keep phone numbers for hospital, doctor, etc. by the telephone.

▶ Make sure friends or family members have your doctor's telephone number.

▶ Instruct friends and family on proper first aid for convulsions and when to call an ambulance.

▶ Consider installing a home security system with a "panic button."

▶ Lay down carpets on all floors.

FIRST AID FOR SEIZURES (SEE CHAPTER 1)

Note: Most seizures are self-limited and require little intervention. Here are some practical guidelines.

What should I do when someone is having a seizure? That question is asked over and over by families and friends of individuals with epilepsy, particularly concerning a tonic–clonic seizure or convulsion. Witnessing a tonic–clonic seizure is an extremely frightening experience. When a seizure occurs, there are few things that an observer can do to help. It is important that fear and frustration do not cause observers to respond in a way that may actually make things worse. The following are a few suggestions about what observers should do during a seizure:

1. **Time the seizure.** This may be important in making the decision as to whether emergency help should be summoned.

2. **Observe the seizure behavior carefully.** This may help the doctor better understand the cause of the seizures and select appropriate medication.

3. **Protect the person having the seizure.** Keep them from falling, hitting their head, or injuring themselves.

4. **Do not put anything in the individual's mouth.** During a seizure, the individual can not breathe well (and may at times appear blue around the lips). After a seizure is over, they will begin to breathe again, but during the seizure there is nothing that an observer can do to help the person breathe. A person having a seizure cannot "swallow their tongue," so there is no need to try to put something into the individual's mouth.

5. **Do not attempt cardiopulmonary resuscitation (CPR) unless the patient stops breathing.** Call for emergency services if jerking movements last longer than 3 minutes.

6. **When possible, roll the patient on his or her side.** This may not be possible during the seizure itself, but should be accomplished as soon as possible. While lying on the side, blood and saliva can more easily drain from the mouth, making it easier for the individual to breath.

7. **After the seizure, clear their airway of saliva, blood, or vomit if possible.**

8. **Allow the person to wake up on his own;** there is no need to stimulate or shake the person who is sleeping after a seizure.

9. **Do not restrain the person,** either during or after the seizure, as this may contribute to more agitation and aggressiveness. You may need to intervene if the individual is going to do something dangerous (such as walking out into traffic).

10. **Stay with the person** until he or she is back to normal level of alertness or until other help arrives.

11. **Notify patient's physician of seizure** and do not allow the patient to drive. Tell the patient what happened.

For Seizures that are not convulsive, the following is helpful:

1. Do not restrain the patient.
2. Protect the patient from wandering or walking into stairs, windows, etc. by gently guiding him or her into a safe area.
3. Do not try to reason with patient during the seizure.
4. Stay with the patient until confusion clears.
5. Notify patient's family, friends and physician of seizure.
6. Do not allow the patient to drive that day.
7. Tell the patient what happened.

Glossary of Terms

Absence Seizures (childhood absence epilepsy; also known as petit mal, true petit mal, or pyknolepsy): A seizure disorder in children between 4 years old and adolescence. There are no warnings prior to attacks. Patients have a sudden change in consciousness, with staring and a blank facial expression, usually lasting less than 15 seconds. The EEG shows a typical pattern. Most patients outgrow these seizures by age 16. Seizures may be provoked by hyperventilation. The electroencephalogram reveals generalized 3-Hz spike and wave.

Atypical Absence Seizure: These seizures last longer than typical absence seizures and are more often accompanied by associated muscle tone changes. The EEG is faster or slower than the EEG seen in typical absence.

Agyria (lissencephaly): A type of cortical dysplasia with inadequate cortical sulcation and gyration. The cortex is smooth and thin, with most of the cortical neurons misplaced in a subcortical layer.

Aicardi Syndrome: This disorder affects only girls. Patients have mental retardation, infantile spasms, missing sections of the corpus callosum, and eye abnormalities. Patients often die early. Spinal bone abnormalities are common. This is a genetic disorder.

Ambulatory EEG: An ambulatory electroencephalogram (EEG) monitoring system that uses digital technology and can record EEG activity at home or in other settings for up to 3 to 4 days.

Astatic Seizure: A seizure that results in a fall. A drop attack that may be due to a tonic, atonic, myoclonic, or partial onset seizure. Astatic seizures are usually seen in those with Lennox-Gastaut syndrome.

Atonic Seizure: A seizure that results in loss of muscle tone. The loss of tone may result in the patient falling to the ground. If less intense, the head may drop. Facial and dental injury is common.

Aura: Although an aura is often thought to be the warning of an impending seizure, it actually represents the beginning of a seizure. What the individual experiences depends on where the seizure starts. The most frequent auras are those seen in temporal lobe epilepsy patients. These auras are described as fear, impending doom, déjà vu, etc.

Automatisms: Abnormal, involuntary, or semipurposeful movements that occur during or after an epileptic seizure, usually associated with memory loss. Patients may smack their lips, swallow, chew, rub their hands, walk, or perform more complex movements such as undressing or speaking words and phrases.

Benign Familial Neonatal Convulsions: Occurring primarily on the second or third day after birth, these clonic seizures are inherited through family members. Relatively few children develop this form of epilepsy.

Benign Rolandic Epilepsy: The most common form of epilepsy found in children. Also known as *benign epilepsy with centrotemporal spikes*, the name refers to electrical discharges seen on the EEG. Seizures begin between the ages of 4 and 13 years. The seizures are characterized by speech arrest, salivation, and facial jerking. Convulsions also may occur. Most of the seizures occur during sleep or soon after waking up. Patients respond well to antiepileptic drugs, but many do not require medication. Benign rolandic epilepsy is age related, and seizures disappear by age 16.

Catamenial Epilepsy: Seizures somehow related to the time of menstruation. The seizures may take place anytime before, during, or after the menstrual period. Approximately half of all women with epilepsy have catamenial seizures.

Clonic Seizure: Repetitive jerking of muscles during a seizure. Most often, clonic seizures start in the upper or lower limb (hand, arm, face, etc). If the seizures follow a pattern of involvement of the hand to the face and the leg they are called Jacksonian seizures (see Introduction).

Computerized Axial Tomography (CAT or CT scan): An imaging technique based on X-ray images taken in different planes by a movable gantry and reconstructed to provide views of the skull and brain. CAT scans are particularly useful when searching for blood, or skull defects but they may not detect small seizure inducing lesions

Convulsion: A generalized tonic–clonic seizure. A partial seizure may spread to become a convulsion, or a convulsion may begin globally without a focal onset.

Corpus Callosotomy: A type of epilepsy surgery particularly used for patients who have "drop attacks" due to atonic seizures and who are at risk for injury. This form of surgery requires splitting the fibers of the corpus callosum, which is the bridge of fibers that connects the right and left half of the brain. Many of these patients have Lennox-Gastaut syndrome. This surgery can greatly reduce drop attacks, but it does not improve partial seizures.

Dysplasia: Abnormal tissue or tissue in the wrong place; usually not tumor related. Dysplasias constitute a large number of disorders that are often associated with childhood epilepsy.

Déjà Vu: A common aura described as having a sensation that a new experience has actually occurred before. A déjà vu sensation may occur as an aura prior to a complex partial or generalized seizure and is most common in temporal lobe epilepsy.

Depth Electrodes: Invasive electrodes used to determine the seizure focus when scalp electroencephalograms remain inconclusive. Typically, four to six electrodes are placed stereotactically into the brain under computed axial tomography or magnetic resonance imaging guidance through small holes drilled into the skull. These electrodes are associated with a small risk of hemorrhage and infection.

Electroencephalogram (EEG): Recording of brain electrical activity. The EEG was discovered by Hans Berger in 1929 and remains an essential component of epilepsy diagnosis and treatment. The EEG is usually recorded with scalp electrodes distributed in an array over the head. The electrical signal is filtered, amplified, and continuously recorded. Typically, 16 channels of electrical activity from different brain areas are displayed. Most EEG recordings take 30 minutes of continuous recording.

Epilepsia Partialis Continua: A form of continuous focal motor seizures, usually of the face or arms, lasting hours, days, or months. These represent simple partial seizures. Most common causes include Rasmussen's encephalitis (see also) and viral diseases.

Epilepsy with Grand Mal Seizures on Awakening: A genetic form of epilepsy with average age of onset at 16 or 17 years. Nearly all convulsions occur after awakening from sleep. Seizures respond well to antiepileptic medication but often recur when drugs are stopped.

Epileptic Syndrome: A group of symptoms and signs, seizure types, cause, genetics, location, age of onset, precipitating factors, and other characteristics. Defining a patient within an epilepsy syndrome guides treatment and improves prognosis. Examples of epilepsy syndromes are benign rolandic epilepsy, childhood absence epilepsy, juvenile myoclonic epilepsy, and West syndrome.

Febrile Seizures: Seizures with fever that occur between the ages of 6 months and 5 years. Most occur during viral infections between 18 and 24 months of age. Very few of these children develop epilepsy. Children with one or two simple febrile seizures do not require chronic antiepileptic drug therapy. These seizures appear to be a benign response to fever that is age related and later outgrown. Children with many febrile seizures are more likely to require ongoing antiepileptic treatment.

Grand Mal Seizures: Convulsive seizures. Loosely translated from French to mean "big bad" seizures. This term is no longer used.

Hemimegalencephaly: One side of the brain is larger than the other. It may be seen in rare developmental cerebral malformations. Usually associated with seizures, developmental delay, and mild weakness of the contralateral (opposite) side of the body.

Hemispherectomy: A type of epilepsy surgery that requires removing or disconnecting the entire or a part of one hemisphere. Many of these patients already have a severe dysfunction of that portion of the brain. Excellent seizure control after this operation is common.

Hertz: A unit of frequency (cycles per second) named after Heinrich Hertz who discovered radio waves.

Heterotopia: A type of malformation in brain development resulting in a cluster of neurons in an abnormal location due to abnormal migration. These misplaced neurons can be the source of epileptic seizures and other neurologic symptoms.

Hippocampal Sclerosis: A loss of neurons and scarring of the hippocampus that is associated with temporal lobe epilepsy. It can appear on magnetic resonance imaging as atrophy and bright spots.

Hippocampus: A portion of the brain responsible for memory function. The structure has the shape of a seahorse and it is often the location of seizures in temporal lobe epilepsy.

Hypsarrhythmia: A dramatic and chaotic pattern on the EEG of patients with infantile spasms. Usually associated with poor response to antiepileptic drugs.

Ictal: "During a seizure." The period of clinical and electrical epileptic activity.

Infantile Spasms (West syndrome): Described in 1841 by West, on observing his own child. Seizures consist of flexor and/or extensor spasms of the body, which tend to occur in clusters. Up to 60% of cases of infantile spasms are associated with strokes, malformations, and other brain lesions. Good outcome is seen in children who are normal when seizures begin and in whom no cause can be found for the spasms.

Interictal: The time between seizures or when patients are not having a seizure. Refers usually to the EEG.

Intractable Epilepsy: A changing definition. In general, seizures that persist despite appropriate treatment. Approximately 35% of patients have seizures that do not respond to adequate doses of appropriate antiepileptic drugs. Patients with intractable epilepsy are candidates for investigational drug trials, epilepsy surgery, and other treatments.

Jamais Vu: A type of aura that is best described as a feeling that a familiar experience has never occurred before (opposite of déjà vu). Jamais vu and déjà vu are types of temporal lobe partial seizures.

Juvenile Myoclonic Epilepsy (Janz syndrome): A primary generalized epilepsy with onset between the ages of 12 and 18 years. Patients have brief jerks (myoclonic seizures) particularly when fatigued. These can occur in clusters and lead to convulsions. Continued treatment is required for most patients.

Ketogenic Diet: A special diet described in the beginning of the 20th century to treat seizures. The ketogenic diet requires a high ratio of fat to carbohydrate and protein. Improvement in seizure control is seen particularly in children when the diet is rigorously followed.

Landau-Kleffner Syndrome: An epilepsy syndrome of unknown cause affecting children. It consists of progressive language problems and an epileptiform EEG. 70% of patients with this syndrome have seizures. Severe behavior problems commonly occur. Outcome is variable, with some children making a complete recovery as adults whereas others do not.

Lennox-Gastaut Syndrome: A childhood epileptic syndrome of intractable epilepsy, mental retardation, and slow spike-and-wave on EEG. Multiple seizure types occur, particularly atypical absence, tonic, and drop attacks. Seizures are extremely difficult to control. In addition to the seizures, most of these children have other neurologic abnormalities.

Mesial Temporal Sclerosis: See Hippocampal Sclerosis.

Monotherapy: The treatment of epilepsy using a single medication rather than a combination. Monotherapy has fewer side effects, simpler dosing, and lower cost.

Myoclonus: Brief motor jerks that may represent epileptic seizures or nonepileptic etiologies. Usually affecting arms and hands. Myoclonus is often reported after awakening. Myoclonus is seen in juvenile myoclonic epilepsy.

Neuronal Migration Disorders: Brain malformations that cause seizures. A number of conditions are classified as migration disorders.

Nonepileptic Seizures (Pseudoseizures, Psychogenic Seizures): These may be events such as tics or strokes that are mistaken as epileptic seizures. More commonly, staring spells, abnormal movements, or convulsions result from psychiatric problems such as conversion disorder or panic attacks. Careful studies are often needed to make a correct diagnosis.

Partial Seizure (Focal Seizures): A seizure that begins in a specific area of the brain. Partial seizures are divided into "simple" and "complex" seizures. Partial seizures are the most common type of seizures in adults.

Partial Complex Seizure: A seizure that causes an alteration of consciousness. Partial complex seizures are sometimes called psychomotor seizures. Automatisms, such as lip smacking, chewing, and swallowing are common. Most patients have no memory of the events.

Partial Simple Seizure: A seizure that does not cause an alteration of consciousness. For example, a seizure that causes hand or arm movements. An epileptic aura, such as a smell, visions, or sound, is also a partial simple seizure.

Petit Mal Seizure: See Absence Epilepsy.

Polycystic Ovary Syndrome: A condition characterized by multiple cysts in the ovaries, increased body hair, acne, weight gain, loss of menstrual cycles, and hormonal disruptions. Polycystic ovary syndrome is seen in women with temporal lobe epilepsy and in those taking Depakote.

Polytherapy: The treatment of epilepsy using multiple medication combinations.

Positron Emission Tomography (PET): A computerized imaging technique that allows imaging of brain metabolism. Usually used prior to surgical interventions. May uncover abnormal areas that magnetic resonance imaging may not detect.

Pseudoseizures: See Nonepileptic Seizures.

Psychomotor Epilepsy: See Temporal Lobe Epilepsy.

Pyknolepsy: An older term for childhood absence epilepsy.

Rasmussen's Encephalitis: A rare inflammatory disease in young patients affecting half of the brain and causing progressive weakening of one side which results in mental decline, and intractable seizures. Traditional treatment has been surgery, but immune therapy has also been helpful.

Single Photon Emission Computed Tomography (SPECT): Nuclear medical imaging technique, which may help determine the area of a seizure focus. The injection is given at the time of seizure and is of use in surgical candidates prior to surgery.

Spike: A specific EEG abnormality associated with epileptic seizures.

Spike-Wave: A specific EEG abnormality associated with epileptic seizures.

Status Epilepticus: Recurrent seizures lasting for 30 minutes or more without recovery. Status epilepticus can be life-threatening and thus is a medical emergency.

Subclinical Seizures (Electrographic Seizures): Electrical seizures that do not have any outward signs, but are visible on the EEG.

Subdural Electrodes: Electrodes used during epilepsy surgery. These electrodes are made of plastic and metal and are placed on the surface of the brain by a neurosurgeon to record electrical activity and assist in the location of the seizure focus before surgery.

Temporal Lobectomy: Refers to a *resection* or removal of a section or entire portion of the temporal lobe. This is the most common operation for seizures.

Tonic: The portion of a seizure during which stiffening of muscles occurs. It is part of a generalized tonic–clonic seizure.

Tuberous Sclerosis: A genetic condition characterized by skin lesions, seizures, and cognitive changes. Behavioral and learning problems are common. The diagnosis is essential for genetic counseling. Patients should have cardiac and renal ultrasounds and an ophthalmologic exams to screen for extraneurologic manifestations.

Vagal Nerve Stimulator (NeuroCybernetic Prosthesis): A battery-powered programmable generator, similar to a cardiac pacemaker, that is implanted in the neck. It sends repeated stimulation via an electrode attached to the left vagus nerve. It may help up to 25% of patients with seizure control.

Wada Test: Also known as Amytal procedure. Pioneered by Jun Wada, a Japanese neurosurgeon. This test evaluates how good memory is and may locate on which side of the brain language is located. This test is done before surgical intervention in select patients.

West Syndrome: See Infantile Spasms.

Adverse Events Profile

During the past 4 weeks, have you had any of the problems or side effects listed below? For each item, if it has always or often been a problem, circle 4; if it has sometimes been a problem circle 3; and so on. Please be sure to answer every item.

	Always or often a problem	Sometimes a problem	Rarely a problem	Never a problem
Unsteadiness	4	3	2	1
Tiredness	4	3	2	1
Restlessness	4	3	2	1
Feelings of aggression	4	3	2	1
Nervousness and/or agitation	4	3	2	1
Headache	4	3	2	1
Hair loss	4	3	2	1
Problems with skin, e.g., acne, rash	4	3	2	1
Double or blurred vision	4	3	2	1
Upset stomach	4	3	2	1
Difficulty in concentration	4	3	2	1
Trouble with mouth or gums	4	3	2	1
Shaky hands	4	3	2	1
Weight gain	4	3	2	1
Dizziness	4	3	2	1
Sleepiness	4	3	2	1
Depression	4	3	2	1
Memory problems	4	3	2	1
Disturbed sleep	4	3	2	1

Please make photocopies for your use when visiting your physician.

Name _____

Year _____

Month _____

SUNDAY	MONDAY	TUESDAY	WEDNESDAY	THURSDAY	FRIDAY	SATURDAY

Please make photocopies for your use when visiting your physician.

INDEX

Note: Boldface numbers indicate illustrations; italic t indicates a table.